Venereal Disease

Bibliography

For

1971

Venereal Disease
Bibliography
For
1971

⌐ ⌐ ⌐

compiled by
Stephen H. Goode

The Whitston Publishing Company
Incorporated
Troy, New York
1973

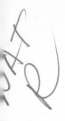

PREFACE

This is the first annual supplement to VENEREAL
DISEASE BIBLIOGRAPHY, 1966-1970, (Whitston, 1972). It
is a near-complete world bibliography of venereal disease literature for 1971. Those entries coming too late
for inclusion in the 1966-1970 volume are entered here;
those too late for this volume will appear in the second
annual supplement.

The following indexes, bibliographies, and abstracts
were searched in the compilation of this bibliography:
APPLIED SCIENCE AND TECHNOLOGY INDEX; BIBLIOGRAPHIC INDEX;
BOOKS IN PRINT; BRITISH HUMANITIES INDEX; BUSINESS PERI-
ODICALS INDEX; CANADIAN PERIODICAL INDEX; CUMULATIVE BOOK
INDEX; CURRENT LITERATURE ON VENEREAL DISEASE; EDUCATION
INDEX; HOSPITAL LITERATURE INDEX; INDEX MEDICUS; INTER-
NATIONAL NURSING INDEX; LIBRARY OF CONGRESS: BOOKS; SUB-
JECTS; NURSING LITERATURE INDEX; PUBLIC AFFAIRS INFOR-
MATION SERVICE; READERS GUIDE TO PERIODICAL LITERATURE;
SOCIAL SCIENCES AND HUMANITIES INDEX.

Although this volume is an attempt at a complete
bibliography of venereal disease per se, it is selective
in such gray areas as trichomoniasis, candidiasis, vaginitis, etc. That is, it does not list entries concerning
Candida which would be of interest only to the researcher
interested in the structure of Candida; but candidiasis

infections, if conceivably of interest to the VD special-
ist or clinician, have been included.

Thus, one will find entries such as "The effect of
cephaloridine and a cephalosporin derivative on mycoplasmas;" but not, for example, an article entitled
"Heterogeneity among strains of mycoplasma granularum and
identification of mycoplasma hyosynoviae," or "Similar-
ities of mycoplasma species isolated from man and from
nonhuman primates."

The arrangement and various qualifications applying
to the basic volume, 1966-1970, also govern the use of
this supplement.

Although there are refinements here over the basic
volume, comments and suggestions for improving the usefulness of this series will be warmly appreciated.

Stephen Goode

LIST OF ABBREVIATIONS
AND PERIODICALS

Abbreviation	Title
Acta Cytol	Acta Cytologica (Baltimore)
Acta Derm Venereol	Acta Dermato-Venereologica (Stockholm)
Acta Med Scand	Acta Medica Scandinavica (Stockholm)
Acta Obstet Gynecol Scand	Acta Obstetricia et Gynecologica Scandinavica (Lund)
Acta Otorinolarynol Iber Am	Acta Oto-Rino-Laryngologica Ibero-Americana (Barcelona)
Acta Paediatr Scand	Acta Paediatrica Scandinavica (Stockholm)
Acta Pathol Microbiol Scand	Acta Pathologica et Microbiologica Scandinavica Section A: Pathology (formerly Acta Pathologica et Microbiologica Scandinavica) Section B: Microbiology and Immunology (Copenhagen)
Acta Vet Scand	Acta Veterinaria Scandinavica (Copenhagen)
Actas Dermosifiliogr	Actas Dermosifiliograficas (Madrid)
Aerosp Med	Aerospace Medicine (St. Paul)
Am Druggist	American Druggist (New York)
Am Fam Physician	American Family Physician (Kansas City, Missouri)
Am J Clin Pathol	American Journal of Clinical Pathology (Baltimore)

Am J Med	American Journal of Medicine (New York)
Am J Med Technol	American Journal of Medical Technology (Houston)
Am J Nurs	American Journal of Nursing (New York)
Am J Obstet Gynecol	American Journal of Obstetrics and Gynecology (St. Louis)
Am J Occup Ther	American Journal of Occupational Therapy (New York)
Am J Ophthamol	American Journal of Ophthalmol (Chicago)
Am J Proctol	American Journal of Proctology (New York)
Am Rev Resp Dis	American Review of Respiratory Disease (Baltimore)
Am J Dis Child	American Journal of Diseases of Children (Chicago)
Amer J Epidemiol	American Journal of Epidemiology (Baltimore)
Anesth Analg	Anesthesia and Analgesia; Current Researches (Cleveland
Ann Allergy	Annals of Allergy (St. Paul)
Ann Biol Clin	Annales de Biologie Clinique (Paris)
Ann Intern Med	Annals of Internal Medicine (Philadelphia)
Ann Med Interne	Annales de Medicine Interne (Paris)
Ann Pharm Fr	Annales Pharmaceutiques Francaises (Paris)
Antimicrob Agents Chemother	Antimicrobial Agents and Chemotherapy (Detroit)
Appl Microbiol	Applied Microbiology (Baltimore.
Arch Biochem Biophys	Archives of Biochemistry and Biophysics (New York)
Arch Dermatol	Archives of Dermatology (Chicago
Arch Hyg Bakteriol	Archiv fur Hygiene und Bakteriologie (Munich)
Arch Intern Med	Archives of Internal Medicine (Chicago)

Arch Mikrobiol	Archiv fur Mikrobiologie (Berlin)
Arch Pathol	Archives of Pathology (Chicago)
Arch Roum Pathol Exp Microbiol	Archives Roumaines de Pathologie Experimentale et de Microbiologie (Bucharest)
Arcisp S Anna Ferrara	Arcispedale S. Anna de Ferrara: Rivista Bimestrale di Scienze Mediche (Ferrara)
Ariz Med	Arizona Medicine (Scottsdale)
Ariz Nurse	Arizona Nurse (Phoenix)
Arthritis Rheum	Arthritis and Rheumatism (New York)
Arzneim Forsch	Arzneimittal-Forschung (Aulendorf)
Aust Vet J	Australian Veterinary Journal (Sydney)
Berufsdernatosen	Berufsdernatosen (Aulendorf)
Biochem Biophys Res Commun	Biochemical and Biophysical Research Communications (New York)
Biochim Biophys Acta	Biochimica et Biophysica Acta (Amsterdam)
Biokhimiia	Biokhimiia (Moscow)
Biotechnol Bioeng	Biotechnology and Bioengineering (New York)
Bol Chil Parasitol	Boletin Chileno de Parasitologia (Santiago)
Bol of Sanit Panama	Boletin de la Oficina Sanitaria Panamericana (Washington)
Bord Med	Bordeaux Medical (Bordeaux)
Br J Dermatol	British Journal of Dermatology (London)
Br J Exp Pathol	British Journal of Experimental Pathology (London)
Br Med J	British Medical Journal (London)
Brain Nerve	Brain and Nerve (Tokyo)
Bratisl Lek Listy	Bratislavske Lekarske Listy (Bratislava)
Brit J Clin Pract	British Journal of Clinical Practice (London)
Brit J Vener Dis	British Journal of Venereal

	Diseases (London)
Brux Med	Bruxelles-Medical (Brussels)
Bull Hist Med	Bulletin of the History of Medicine (Baltimore)
Bull Hosp Joint Dis	Bulletin of the Hospital for Joint Diseases (New York)
Bull Ophthalmol Soc Egypt	Bulletin of the Ophthalmologica Society of Egypt (Cairo)
Bull Soc Fr Dermatol Syphiligr	Bulletin de la Societe Fran-caise de Dermatologie et de Syphiligraphie (Paris)
Bull Soc Ophthalmol Fr	Bulletin des Societes d'Ophthal mologie de France (Paris)
Bull Soc Pathol Exot	Bulletin de la Societe de Pathologie Exotique et de ses Filiales (Paris)
C R Acad Sci	Comptes Rendus Herdomadaires des Seances de l'Academie des Sciences; D: Sciences Naturelles (Paris)
Calif Med	California Medicine (San Fran-cisco)
Can J Med Technol	Canadian Journal of Medical Technology (Hamilton)
Can J Microbiol	Canadian Journal of Microbio-logy (Ottawa)
Can J Public Health	Canadian Journal of Public Heal (Toronto)
Can Nurse	Canadian Nurse (Ottawa)
Cancer	Cancer (Philadelphia)
Cas Lek Cesk	Casopis Lekaru Ceskych (Prague)
Cent Afr J Med	Central Africa Journal of Medi-cine (Salisbury)
Cesk Dermatol	Ceskoslovenska Dermatologie (Prague)
Cesk Epidemiol Mikrobiol Imunol	Ceskoslovenska Epidemiologie, Mikrobiologie, Imunologie (Prague)
Cesk Pediatr	Ceskoslovenska Pediatrie (Pragu
Cesk Psychiatr	Ceskoslovenska Psychiatrie (Prague)

Chem & Eng N	Chemical and Engineering News (Washington)
Clin Obstet Gynecol	Clinical Obstetrics and Gynecology (New York)
Clin Pediatr	Clinical Pediatrics (Philadelphia)
Clin Symposia	Clinical Symposia (Summit, New Jersey)
Coeur Med Interne	Coeur et Medecine Interne (Paris)
Current Dig Soviet Pr	Current Digest of the Soviet Press (Columbus)
Disease-A-Month	Disease-A-Month (Chicago)
Dent Stud	Dental Student (Northfield, Illinois)
Dermatologica	Dermatologica (Basel)
Dis Colon Rectum	Diseases of the Colon and Rectum (Philadelphia)
Dtsch Gesundheitsw	Deutsche Gesundheitswesen (Berlin)
Dtsch Med Wochenschr	Deutsch Medizinische Wochenschrift (Stuttgart)
Duodecim	Duodecim (Helsinki)
East Africa Med J	East African Medical Journal (Nairobi)
Electroencephalogr Clin Neurophysiol	Electroencephalography and Clinical Neurophysiology (Amsterdam)
Emergency Med	Emergency Medicine (New York)
Ethiop Med J	Ethiopian Medical Journal (Addis Ababa)
Feldsher Akush	Fel'dsher i Akusherka (Moswow)
Folia Med	Folia Medica (Naples); Folia Medica (Plovidiv)
Folia Microbiol	Folia Microbiologica (Prague)
Forecast Home Econ	Forecast for Home Economics (New York)
Fortschr Geb Roetgenstr Nuklearmed	Fortschritte auf dem Gebiete der Roentgenstrahlen und der Nuklearmedizin (Stuttgart)
Gac Med Mex	Gaceta Medica de Mexico (Mexico City)

Ginecol Obstet Mex	Ginecologia y Obstetricia de Mexico (Mexico City)
G Ital Dermatol	Giornale Italiano di Dermatologia-Minerva Dermatologica (Turin)
Geburtshilfe Frauenheilkd	Geburtshilfe und Frauenheilkunde (Stuttgart)
Gynaekol Rundsch	Gynaekologische Rundschau (Base
Gynecol Prat	Gynecologie Pratique (Paris)
HSMHA Health Rep	HSMHA Health Reports (Washington)
Harefuah	Harefuah (Tel Aviv)
Hautarzt	Hautarzt (Berlin)
Health Lab Sci	Health Laboratory Science (New York)
Hoppe Seylers Z Physiol Chem	Hoppe-Seyler's Zeitschrift fur Physiologische Chemie (Berlin
Hosp Pract	Hospital Practice (New York)
Hospital	Hospital (Rio de Janiero)
Humanist	Humanist (London, Utrecht, Amherst, Massachusetts)
Indian J Dermatol	Indian Journal of Dermatology (Calcutta)
Infirm Fr	L'Infirmiere Francaise (Paris)
Int Arch Allergy Appl Immunol	International Archives of Allergy and Applied Immunology (Basel)
Int J Dermatol	International Journal of Dermatology (Philadelphia)
Int Z Klin Pharmacol Ther Toxikol	Internationale Zeitschrift fur Kinische Pharmakologie, Therapie und Toxikologie (Munich)
Invest Urol	Investigative Urology (Baltimore)
Isr J Med Sci	Israel Journal of Medical Sciences (Jerusalem)
JAMA	Journal of the American Medical Association (Chicago)
J Allergy	Journal of Allergy (St. Louis)
J Am Osteopath Assoc	Journal of the American Osteo-

	pathic Association (Chicago)
J Antibiot	Journal of Antibiotics (Tokyo)
J Bacteriol	Journal of Bacteriology (Baltimore)
J Bone Joint Surg	Journal of Bone and Joint Surgery; American volume (Boston); British volume (London)
J Cardiovasc Surg	Journal of Cardiovascular Surgery (Turin)
J Chir	Journal de Chirurgie (Paris)
J Chromatogr	Journal of Chromatography (Amsterdam)
J Chronic Dis	Journal of Chronic Diseases (St. Louis)
J Clin Pathol	Journal of Clinical Pathology (London)
J Immunol	Journal of Immunology (Baltimore)
J Indian Med Assoc	Journal of the Indian Medical Association (Calcutta)
J Indiana State Med Assoc	Journal of the Indiana State Medical Association (Indianapolis)
J Infect Dis	Journal of Infectious Diseases (Chicago)
J Iowa Med Soc	Journal of the Iowa Medical Society (Des Moines)
J Jap Assoc Infect Dis	Journal of the Japanese Association for Infectious Disease (Tokyo) in Japanese: Kansenshogaku Zasshi
J Kans Med Soc	Journal of the Kansas Medical Society (Topeka)
J La State Med Soc	Journal of the Louisiana State Medical Society (New Orleans)
J Lab Clin Med	Journal of Laboratory and Clinical Medicine (St. Louis)
J Laryngol Otol	Journal of Laryngology and Otology (London)
J Med Assoc State Ala	Journal of the Medical Association of the State of Alabama

ix

	(Montgomery)
J Med Assoc Thai	Journal of the Medical Association of Thailand (Bangkok)
J Med Lyon	Journal de Medecine de Lyon (Lyon)
J Med Microbiol	Journal of Medical Microbiology (Edinburgh)
J Natl Med Ass	Journal of the National Medical Association (New York)
J Okla State Med Ass	Journal of the Oklahoma State Medical Association (Oklahoma City)
J Parasitol	Journal of Parasitology (Chicag◖
J Pathol	Journal of Pathology (London)
J Pediatr	Journal of Pediatrics (St. Loui
J Pract Nurs	Journal of Practical Nursing (New York)
J Sch Health	Journal of School Health (Colum◖ bus)
J Sci Med Lille	Journal des Sciences Medicales de Lille (Lille)
J Tenn Med Assoc	Journal of the Tennessee Medica. Association (Nashville)
J Urol	Journal of Urology (Baltimore)
Jap Circ J	Japanese Circulation Journal (Kyoto)
Jap Heart J	Japanese Heart Journal (Tokyo)
Jap J Physiol	Japanese Journal of Physiology (Kyoto)
Johns Hopkins Med J	Johns Hopkins Medical Journal (Baltimore)
Lakartidningen	Lakartidningen (Stockholm)
Lancet	Lancet (London)
Listener	Listener (London)
Lyon Med	Lyon Medical (Lyon)
McCalls	McCalls (New York)
Maroc Med	Maroc Medical (Casablanca)
Mars Med	Marseille Medical (Marseille)
Med Ann DC	Medical Annals of the District of Columbia (Washington)
Med Dosw Mikrobiol	Medycyna Doswiadczalna i Mikro-

	biologia (Warsaw)
Med J Aust	Medical Journal of Australia (Sydney)
Med Klin	Medizinische Klinik (Munich)
Med Lett Drugs Ther	Medical Letter on Drugs and Therapeutics (New York)
Med Parazitol	Meditsinskaia Parazitologiia i Parazitarnye Bolezni (Moscow)
Med Times	Medical Times (Manhasset)
Med Welt	Medizinische Welt (Stuttgart)
Med World News	Medical World News (New York)
Mich Med	Michigan Medicine (East Lansing)
Microbiol, Parazitol, Epidemiol	Microbiologia, Parazitologia, Epidemiologia (Bucharest)
Midwife Health Visit	Midwife and Health Visitor (London)
Mikrobiol Zh	Mikrobiolohichnyi Zhurnal (Kiev)
Minerva Ginecol	Minerva Ginecologica (Turin)
Mo Med	Missouri Medicine (St. Paul)
Munca Sanit	Munca Sanitara Nursing Care (Bucharest)
Munch Med Wochenschr	Muenchener Medizinische Wochenschrift (Munich)
Mycopathol Mycol Appl	Mycopathologia et Mycologie Applicata (The Hague)
Mykosen	Mykosen (Berlin)
N Engl J Med	New England Journal of Medicine (Boston)
NY State Ed	New York State Education (Albany)
NY State J Med	New York State Journal of Medicine (New York)
NY Times Mag	New York Times Magazine (New York)
NZ Med J	New Zealand Medical Journal (Wellington)
Naika	Naika (Tokyo)
Nature	Nature (London)
Naturwissenschaften	Naturwissenschaften (Berlin)
Ned Tijdschr Geneeskd	Nederlands Tijdschrift voor Geneeskunde (Amsterdam)
Neurochirurgia	Neurochirurgia (Stuttgart)

Neurol Neurochir Pol	Neurologia i Neurochirurgia Polska (Warsaw)
Neuropatol Pol	Neuropatologia Polska (Warsaw)
Neuropsihijatrija	Neuropsihijatrija (Zagreb)
Newsweek	Newsweek (New York)
Niger Nurse	Nigerian Nurse (Lagos)
Nord Med	Nordisk Medicin (Stockholm)
Northwest Med	Northwest Medicine (Seattle)
Nurs Mirror	Nursing Mirror and Midwives' Journal (London)
Nurs Times	Nursing Times (London)
Observer	Observer (London)
Obstet Gynecol	Obstetrics and Gynecology (New York)
Occup Health	Occupational Health (Auckland)
Orv Hetil	Orvosi Hetilap (Budapest)
Otorinolaringologie	Oto-Rino-Laringologie (Bucharest
Pathol Biol	Pathologie et Biologie (Paris)
Pathol Vet	Pathologia Veterinaria (Basel)
Pediatr Pol	Pediatria Polska (Warsaw)
Pediatr Akush Ginekol	Pediatriia Akusherstvo i Ginekologiia (Kiev)
Pediatrics	Pediatrics (Springfield, Illinoi
Pediatrie	Pediatrie (Bucharest)
Pieleg Polozna	Pielegniarka i Polozna (Warsaw)
Pol Med J	Polish Medical Journal (Warsaw)
Pol Przegl Chir	Polski Przeglad Chirurgiczny (Warsaw)
Pol Tyg Lek	Polski Tygodnik Lekarski (Warsaw
Policlinico	Policlinico; Sezione Pratica (Rome)
Postgrad Med J	Postgraduate Medical Journal (London)
Practitioner	Practitioner (London)
Praxis	Praxis (Bern)
Prensa Med Argent	Prensa Medica Argentina (Buenos Aires)
Presse Med	Presse Medicale (Paris)
Probl Gematol Pereliv Krove	Problemy Gematologii i Pere-livaniia Krovi (Moscow)
Proc R Soc Med	Proceedings of the Royal Society

	of Medicine (London)
Przegl Dermatol	Przeglad Dermatologieczny (Warsaw)
Przegl Epidemiol	Przeglad Epidemiologiczny (Warsaw)
Przegl Lek	Przeglad Lekarski (Krakow)
Public Health	Public Health (London)
R Soc Health J	Royal Society of Health Journal (London)
Radiology	Radiology (Syracuse)
Rev Bras Med	Revista Brasileira de Medicina (Rio de Janiero)
Rev Colomb Obstet Ginecol	Revista Colombiana de Obstetricia y Gynecologia (Bogota)
Rev Fr Allergol	Revue Francaise d'Allergologie (Paris)
Rev Inst Med Trop Sao Paulo	Revista do Instituto de Medicina Tropical de Sao Paulo (Sao Paulo)
Rev Med Chil	Revista Medica de Chile (Santiago)
Rev Otoneuroophtalmol	Revue d'oto-neuro-ophtalmologie (Paris)
Rev Paul Med	Revista Paulista de Medicina (Sao Paula)
Rev Saude Publica	Revista de Saude Publica (Sao Paulo)
Rocky Mtn Med J	Rocky Mountain Medical Journal (Denver)
Rom Med Rev	Romanian Medical Review (Bucharest)
S Afr Med J	South Africian Medical Journal (Capetown)
Sabouraudia	Sabouraudia (Edinburgh)
Saishin Igaku	Saishin Igaku (Osaka)
Salud Publica Mex	Salud Publica de Mexico (Mexico City)
Sanfujinka Jissai	Sanfujinka no Jissai (Tokyo)
Scand J Infect Dis	Scandinavian Journal of Infectious Diseases (Stockholm)
Science	Science (Washington)

Semin Hematol	Seminars in Hematology (New York)
Soc Sci Med	Social Science and Medicine (Oxford)
South Med J	Southern Medical Journal (Birmingham)
Stomatologiia	Stomatologiia (Moscow)
Texas Med	Texas Medicine (Austin)
Tidsskr Nor Laegeforen	Tidsskrift for den Norske Laegeforening (Oslo)
Times Educ Sup	Times Educational Supplement (London)
Todays Educ	Todays Education (Washington)
Today's Health	Today's Health (Chicago)
Trans R Soc Trop Med Hyg	Transactions of the Royal Socie of Tropical Medicine and Hygiene (London)
Trop Geogr Med	Tropical and Geographical Medicine (Haarlem)
Ugeskr Laeger	Ugeskrift for Laeger (Copenhagen)
Va Med Mon	Virginia Medical Monthly (Richmond)
Vestn Akad Med Nauk SSSR	Vestnik Akademii Nauk SSSR (Moscow)
Vestn Dermatol Venerol	Vestnik Dermatologii i Venerologii (Moscow)
Voen Med Zh	Voenno-Meditsinskii Zhurnal (Moscow)
Vopr Okhr Materin Det	Voprosy Okhrany Materinstva i Detstva (Moscow)
Vrach Delo	Vrachebnoe Delo (Kiev)
WHO Chron	WHO Chronical (Geneva)
Wiad Parazytol	Wiadomosci Parazytologiczne (Warsaw)
Wien Klin Wochenschr	Wiener Klinische Wochenschrift (Vienna)
Wien Med Wochenschr	Wiener Medizinische Wochenschrift (Vienna)
Wis Med J	Wisconsin Medical Journal (Madison)
World Health	World Health (Geneva)

Z Allg Mikrobiol	Zeitschrift fur Allgemeine Mikrobiologie (Berlin)
Z Allgemeinmed	Zeitschrift fur Allgemeinmedizin: der Landarzt (Stuttgart)
Z Haut Geschlechtskr	Zeitschrift fur Haut- und Geschlechts-Krankheiten (Berlin)
Z Immunitaetsforsch Allerg Klin Immunol	Zeitschrift fur Immunitaetsforschung, Allergie und Klinische Immunologie (Stuttgart)
Z Orthop	Zeitschrift fur Orthopaedie und Ihre Grenzgebiete (Stuttgart)
Z Tropenmed Parasitol	Zeitschrift fur Tropenmediain und Parasitologie (Stuttgart)
Zentralbl Allg Pathol	Zentralblatt fur Allgemeine Pathologie und Pathologische Anatomie (Jena)
Zentralbl Bakteriol	Zentralblatt fur Bakteriologie, Parasitenkunde, Infektionskrankheiten und Hygiene: Erste Abteiling: Originale (Stuttgart)
Zentralbl Gynaekol	Zentralblatt fur Gynaekologie (Leipzig)
Zh Mikrobiol Epidemiol Immunobiol	Zhurnal Mikrobiologii, Epidemiologii i Immunobiologii (Moscow)
Zh Nevropathol Psikhiatr	Zhurnal Nevropatologii i Psikhiatrii Imeni S. S. Korsakove (Moscow)

SUBJECT HEADINGS USED IN THIS BIBLIOGRAPHY

American Medical Association
Amphotericin B
Ampicillin
Ano-Rectal Venereal Diseases
Arthritis
Balanitis and Balanoposthitis
Bay B 5097
Bedsoniae
Beethoven's Disease
Bejel
Bicillin
Biotin
Blennorrhagia
Blood Donors and Transfus-
  ions
Cancer and Pre-Cancer
Candida and Candidiasis
Candicidin
Candidine
Candistatin
Carbenoxolone
Cephalexin
Cephalosporins
Chancroid
Children
Chloromycetin
College Students and VD
Colpitis
Contraception and Contra-
  ceptives

Copiamycin
Corticosteroids
DNA
Dentistry
Detreomycin
Diagnosis
Doxycycline
Drug Addiction
Education
Epididymitis
Erythromycin
Fertility, Infertility, and
  Sterility
Flagyl
Gentamycin
Gonorrhea
Gonorrhea: Ano-Rectal
Gonorrhea: Arthritic
Gonorrhea: Cerebro-Spinal
Gonorrhea: Children
Gonorrhea: Complications
Gonorrhea: Diagnosis
Gonorrhea: Hepatic
Gonorrhea: Naso-Pharynegeal
Gonorrhea: Neonatal
Gonorrhea: Occurrence
Gonorrhea: Ophthalmic
Gonorrhea: Penile

TABLE OF CONTENTS

BOOKS

Bender, Stephen J. VENEREAL DISEASE. Dubuque, Iowa:
   W. C. Brown Company, 1971.

Clowes, William. BOOKE OF OBSERVATIONS. Amsterdam:
   Theatrum Orbis Terrarum; New York: Da Capo Press,
   1971.

Darrow, William W. SELECTED REFERENCES ON THE BEHAV-
   IORAL ASPECTS OF VENEREAL DISEASE CONTROL; an anno-
   tated bibliography for behavioral scientists, epidem-
   iologists, and venereal disease casefinding personnel.
   Atlanta: Center for Disease Control, 1971.

Dethmers, P. DERMATOLOGIE EN VENEROLOGIE; EEN INLEIDING
   VOOR MEDISCHE STUDENTEN EN VERPLEEGKUNDIGN. Lochem:
   De Tijdstroom, 1971.

Grover, John W. VD: THE ABC'S. Englewood Cliffs, New
   Jersey: Prentice-Hall, 1971.

Rosebury, Theodor. MICROBES AND MORALS: THE STRANGE
   STORY OF VENEREAL DISEASE. New York: Viking, 1971.

PERIODICAL LITERATURE

TITLE INDEX

"AMA statement on venereal disease." MO MED. 68:604, August, 1971.

"APP treats gonorrhea." AM DRUGGIST. 163:46, May 3, 1971.

"Abnormal chemoreceptor response to hypoxia in patients with tabes dorsalis," by R. J. Evans, et al. BR MED J. 1:530-531, March 6, 1971.

"About a new medium for culture of Trichomonas vaginalis," by N. Jankov, et al. FOLIA MED. 13:137-140, 1971.

"Achievements in the control of dermatologic and venereal diseases in Yamal (40th anniversary of the formation of the Yamal-Nenets National Region)," by N. A. Belonogova, et al. VESTN DERMATOL VENEROL. 45:61-63, June, 1971.

"Achievements in dermatovenereology in Georgia (1921-1971)," by L. T. Shetsiruli, et al. VESTN DERMATOL VENEROL. 45:72-76, November, 1971.

"Acquired syphilis--drugs and blood tests," by W. J. Brown. AMER J NURS. 71:713-715, April, 1971.

"Action of Nifuratel on lower genital infections," by M. Fayette. J MED LYON. 52:1445-1451, November 5, 1971.

"Acute choroido-retinitis in secondary syphillis. Presence of spiral organisms in the aqueous humour," by P. A. Macfaul, et al. BR J VENER DIS. 47:159-161, June, 1971.

"Acute disseminated and chronic mucocutaneous candidiasis," by P. G. Quie, et al. SEMIN HEMATOL. 8:227-242, July, 1971.

"Acute gonococcal perihepatitis (Fitz-Hugh-Curtis syndrome). An acute, right-side 'pleuritic-peritonitic' upper abdominal pain syndrome in Adnexitis gonorrhoica: diagnosis by laparoscopy," by R. Amman, et al. DTSCH MED WOCHENSCHR. 96:1515-1519, September 24, 1971.

"Acute hypersensitivity reaction to penicillin during general anesthesia: a case report," by D. R. Cook, et al. ANESTH ANALG. 50:152-155, January-February, 1971.

"Adequate treatment for syphillis," by G. Allyn. ARCH DERMATOL. 103:462, April, 1971.

"Administration of oxytetracycline hydrochloride with hydrocortisone (Oxycort aerosol) in the treatment of non-specific vaginitis," by A. Ostrzeński. POL TYG LEK. 26:283-284, February 22, 1971.

"Advances in the study of venereal disease," by A. J. King. BR J CLIN PRACT. 25:295-301, July, 1971.

"Advances in the treatment of sexually transmitted diseases," by R. D. Catterall. PRACTITIONER. 207:516-523, October, 1971.

Albert Neisser (1855-1916)," by H. Schwarz. INVEST UROL. 8:478-480, January, 1971.

"Alkane oxidation by a particulate preparation from Candida," by C. M. Liu, et al. J BACTERIOL. 106:830-834, June, 1971.

4

"Alternate methods of nutrient dosing in continuous phased culture," by P. S. Dawson, et al. CAN J MICROBIOL. 17:435-439, April, 1971.

"Amino acid composition of treponemes," by C. W. Moss, et al. BR J VENER DIS. 47:165-168, June, 1971.

"Ampicillin in the treatment of gonorrheal salpingitis," by E. Hedberg, et al. LAKARTIDNINGEN. 68:335-340, January 20, 1971.

"Ampicillin rashes in glandular fever," by H. Pullen. BR MED J. 2:653, June 12, 1971.

"Anal soft chancre and concomitant gonorrhea," by J. Rivoire. BULL SOC FR DERMATOL SYPHILIGR. 78:203, 1971.

"Anal venereal diseases in two practices," by J. Rivoire, et al. AM J PROCTOL. 22:189-190, June, 1971.

"Analysis of early syphilis incidence in the rural environment of the Bialystok province between 1965 and 1969," by H. Szarmach, et al. PRZEGL DERMATOL. 58:279-286, May-June, 1971.

"Analysis of hospital admission rates of patients with syphilis of the central nervous system in Poland before and after World War II," by A. Dowzenko, et al. POL MED J. (Warsaw). 10:539-546, 1971.

"Anaphylactic reaction to oral penicillin," by J. P. Geyman. CALIF MED. 114:87-89, May, 1971.

"Anaphylactic reaction after oral penicillin medication." TIDSSKR NOR LAEGEFOREN. 91:213-214, January 30, 1971.

"Anatomical evidence of pre-columbian syphilis in the West Indian Islands," by N. G. Gejvall, et al. AM J OCCUP THER. 25:138-157, October, 1971.

"Antibiotic-resistant forms of gonorrheal infection,"

by F. V. Potapnev. VESTN DERMATOL VENEROL. 45:51-52, 1971.

"Antibiotics in mycoplasma media and the temporary storage of specimens containing mycoplasmas of the genital tract," by C. S. Goodwin, et al. J CLIN PATHOL. 24:286-287, April, 1971.

"Antibodies binding the complement with antigens of viruses of the ornithosis-psittacosis-lymphogranuloma venereum group and neorickettsiae in various population groups and domestic animals," by C. Frygin, et al. PRZEGL EPIDEMIOL. 25:55-62, 1971.

"Antibodies to gonococcal lipopolysaccharides in patients with gonorrhoea," by M. E. Ward, et al. J MED MOCROBIOL. 4:2-3, May, 1971.

"Antimicrobial activity of sodium n-alkylsalicylates," by D. Buckley, et al. APPL MICROBIOL. 21:565-568, April, 1971.

"Antimicrobial properties of oprophenon," by M. M. Rotmistrov, et al. MIKROBIOL ZH. 33:117-119, 1971.

"Aortic rupture secondary to a suprasigmoid syphilitic gumma. Aortic insufficiency and fatal hemopericardium," by P. Louis, et al. COEUR MED INTERNE. 10:313-321, April-June, 1971.

"Apparent transient false-positive FTA-ABS test following smallpox vaccination." J OKLA STATE MED ASSOC. 64: 372, September, 1971.

"Application of the semi-automatic disposable tip pipette to routine serological test," by P. K. Carter, et al. AM J MED TECHNOL. 37:87-89, March, 1971.

"Apropos of 2 cases of auricular syphilis," by E. Poilpre, et al. REV OTONEUROOPHTALMOL. 43:136-140, April, 1971.

6

"Army treatment of gonorrhea," by J. B. Grossman. ANN INTERN MED. 75:135-136, July, 1971.

"Arthritis, vaginitis and cardiac murmur," by S. Jacobs. J LA STATE MED SOC. 123:179-182, May, 1971.

"An assessment of the role of Candida albicans and food yeasts in chronic urticaria," by J. James, et al. BR J DERMATOL. 84:227-237, March, 1971.

"Attempts to adapt Entamoeba histolytica to various protozoan species on Diamond's TTY medium," by A. Westphal, et al. Z TROPENMED PARASITOL. 22:149-156, June, 1971.

"Attitudes of hospitals in London to venereal disease in the 18th and 19th centuries," by M. A. Waugh. BR J VENER DIS. 47:146-150, April, 1971.

"Atypical case of gonococcal bacteremia," by M. Jacobsen, et al. UGESKR LAEGER. 133:6-7, January 8, 1971.

"Atypical FTA-ABS test fluorescence in lupus erythematosus," by F. Jennis. JAMA. 215:488-489, January 18, 1971.

"Atypical FTA-ABS test reaction. An initial clue in the diagnosis of lupus erythematosus," by S. J. Kraus, et al. ARCH DERMATOL. 104:260-261, September, 1971.

"Atypical fluorescence in the fluorescent treponemal-antibody-absorption (FTA-ABS) test related to deoxyribonucleic acid (DNA) antibodies," by S. J. Kraus, et al. J IMMUNOL. 106:1665-1669, June, 1971.

"Atypical gonorrhoea." BR MED J. 3:322, August 7, 1971.

"Atypical gonorrhoea," by J. Vahrman. BR MED J. 3:579-580, September 4, 1971.

"Autoimmune processes in neuropsychic diseases," by S. F. Semenov. VESTN AKAD MED NAUK SSSR. 26:78-81,

7

1971.

"An automated complement fixation procedure for detecting
    antibody to N. gonorrhoeae," by W. L. Peacock, Jr.
    HSMHA HEALTH REP. 86:706-710, August, 1971.

"The Automated Reagin Test (ART) for syphilis in a pub-
    lic health laboratory," by B. S. West, et al. HEALTH
    LAB SCI. 8:220-224, October, 1971.

"Automated Reagin Test for syphilis in a multichannel
    blood grouping machine," by A. L. Schroeter, et al.
    AM J CLIN PATHOL. 56:43-49, July, 1971.

"Automatic indirect immunofluorescence applied to syphi-
    lis serology (AFTA)," by S. S. Kasatiya, et al. CAN
    J PUBLIC HEALTH. 62:166-168, March-April, 1971.

"Automation of the Wassermann complement-fixation test
    using a discrete analyser," by J. H. Glenn. et al.
    BR J VENER DIS. 47:200-203, June, 1971.

"Bacteria, viruses, and mycoplasmas in acute pneumonia
    in adults," by F. R. Fekety, Jr., et al. AM REV
    RESP DIS. 104:499-507, October, 1971.

"Bacterial hitch-hikers," by T. L. Howard. J UROL. 106:
    94, July, 1971.

"Bactrim (trimethoprim-sulfamethoxazole) treatment of
    female blennorrhagia," by C. B. Schofield, et al.
    REV COLOMB OBSTET GINECOL. 22:269-273, July-August,
    1971.

"Balanitis due to fixed drug eruption associated with
    tetracycline therapy," by G. W. Csonka, et al. BR
    J VENER DIS. 47:42-44, February, 1971.

"Basic results of scientific research on the problem of
    scientific bases of dermatology and venereology for

1969," by N. M. Turanov, et al. VESTN DERMATOL
VENEROL. 44:7-13, September, 1970.

"Bay B 5097, a new orally applicable antifungal sub-
stance with broadspectrum activity. Preliminary clinical and laboratory experiences in children," by W.
Marget, et al. ACTA PAEDIATR SCAND. 60:341-345,
May, 1971.

"Beethoven's disease," by K. Herrero Duclaux. PRENSA
MED ARGENT. 57:2018-2025, January 1, 1971.

"Bejel or non-venereal endemic syphilis," by M. W. Kanan,
et al. BR J DERMATOL. 84:461-464, May, 1971.

"Better specimens from the female genital tract," by S.
Selwyn, et al. BR MED J. 4:170, October 16, 1971.

"Bicillin-6 therapy of gonorrhea in men," by V. E. Grigoriev, et al. VESTN DERMATOL VENEROL. 45:74-77,
January, 1971.

"Birth weight and genital mycoplasmas in pregnancy,"
by P. Braun, et al. N ENGL J MED, 284:167-171,
January 28, 1971.

"'Blitz' proves effective public health tool," by C. F.
Jacobs, et al J LA STATE MED SOC. 123:417 passim,
September, 1971.

"Blood level studies on the depot effect of clemizole-
penicillin G in antiluetic therapy," by D. Kleinhans. Z HAUT GESCHLECHTSKR. 46:359-365, June 1, 1971.

"Blood penicillin levels in patients with gonorrhea
treated according to various therapeutic schedules,"
by J. Bowszyc, et al. PRZEGL DERMATOL. 58:595-599,
September-October, 1971.

"Blood platelet behaviour in syphilis," by S. F. Szanto."
BR J VENER DIS. 47:14-16, February, 1971.

"Brucellosis and syphilis transmitted by transfusion,"
by A. Becerra-García. GAC MED MEX. 101:699-701,
June, 1971.

"CBC done-no VDRL-results: two congenital syphilitics,"
by H. P. Hines, et al. JAP J PHYSIOL. 67:309-310,
July, 1971.

"Can we prevent heart disease?" by L. Werkö. ANN INTERN
MED. 74:278-288, February, 1971.

"Candida and candidiasis," by P. J. Kozinn, et al. JAMA.
217:965-966, August 16, 1971.

"Candida at Boston City Hospital. Clinical and epidemiological characteristics and susceptibility to eight
antimicrobial agents," by P. Toala, et al. ARCH INTER
MED. 126:983-989, December, 1970.

"Candidiasis: colonization vs infection." JAMA. 215:
285-286, January 11, 1971.

"A canine venereal tumor with metastasis to the brain,"
by E. W. Adams, et al. PATHOL VET. 7:498-502, 1970.

"Carbohydrate fermentation patterns of Neisseria meningitidis determined by a microtiter method," by J. A.
Davies, et al. APPL MICROBIOL. 21:1072-1074, June,
1971.

"Case of balanoposthitis trichomonadosa," by Z. Gwieźd-
zinski, et al. POL TYG LEK. 26:642-643, April 26,
1971.

"Case of cerebral gumma of the left temporal lobe," by
K. Kinoshita. BRAIN NERVE. 23:365-368, April, 1971.

"A case of combined inflammatory rheumatic and neuro-
pathic joint changes," by O. Erhart, et al. Z ORTHOP.
107:676-682, May, 1970.

"Case of congenital neurosyphilis with a picture of
juvenile progressive paralysis," by W. Nyka. NEURO-
PATOL POL. 9:353-357, October-December, 1971.

"A case of failure in the treatment of early syphilis
with erythromycin," by Z. Dratwiński. PRZEGL DER-
MATOL. 58:69-71, January-February, 1971.

"Case of gonnorrheic inflamation of the prepuce with negative findings on gonococci in the urethra," by A.
Wierer, et al. CESK DERMATOL. 46:253-255, December,
1971.

"A case of historical syphilis," by F. X. Carton, et al.
BULL SOC FR DERMATOL SYPHILIGR. 78:284-285, 1971.

"A case of juvenile angina pectoris probably due to
congenital syphilis," by T. Kobayashi, et al. JAP
CIRC J. 35:221-226, February, 1971.

"A case of mycosis fungoides (in lues latens seroposi-
tiva) with radiographically detectable pulmonary
granulomas," by H. Standau, et al. Z HAUT GESCH-
LECHTSKR. 46:379-385, June 15, 1971.

"Case of progressive course of tabes dorsalis despite
penicillin treatment and disappearance of changes in
cerebrospinal fluid," by H. Wisniewski, et al. NEUROL
NEUROCHIR POL. 5:237-239, 1971.

"A case of sero-positive primary syphilis of the tonsil,"
by N. H. Vincenti. J LARYNGOL OTOL. 85:869-870,
August, 1971.

"Case of syphilis of the lung," by K. B. Ruszel. POL TYG
LEK. 26:645-646, April 26, 1971.

"A case of syphilitic aneurysum of the aortic sinus and
aortic regurgitation," by S. Okawa, et al. JAP HEART
J. 12:105-110, January, 1971.

"Case report of student aviator with unusual psychoso-

matic symptoms," by J. R. Anderson. AEROSP MED.
42:1217-1218, November, 1971.

"Cell-mediated immunity and lymphocyte transformation
in syphilis," by G. M. Levene, et al. PROC R SOC
MED. 64:426-428, April, 1971.

"Cephalosporin antibiotics in venereal disease," by W.
C. Duncan, et al. POSTGRAD MED J. 47:119-122,
February, 1971.

"Changes in phosphorus composition of Candida utilis
during the cell cycle and postcycle period," by H.
Glättli, et al. CAN J MICROBIOL. 17:339-345, March,
1971.

"Changes in the serum transaminases in patients with
syphilis," by B. S. Tio, et al. BR J VENER DIS. 47:
263-265, August, 1971.

Changes in the trends in syphilis in pregnancy," by C.
Sawazaki, et al. SANFUJINKA JISSAI. 20:112-119,
February, 1971.

"Characteristics of current latent syphilis," by T. V.
Vasil'ev, et al. VESTN DERMATOL VENEROL. 45:45-50,
July, 1971.

"Characteristics of fluorescein labelled antiglobulin
preparations that may affect the fluorescent treponemal antibody-absorption test," by P. H. Hardy, et
al. AM J CLIN PATHOL. 56:181-186, August, 1971.

"A chemically definable enricher of culture media for
Neisseria gonorrhoeae. CESK DERMATOL. 46:23-25,
February, 1971.

"Chemistry of axial filaments of Treponema zuezerae,"
by M. A. Bharier, et al. J BACTERIOL. 105:422-
429, January, 1971.

"Chemotherapeutic activity of liutenurin in experiment-

al trichomoniasis of white mice," by M. A. Rubinchik, et al. MED PARAZITOL. 40:197-201, March-
April, 1971.

"Chlormycetin failure in gonorrhea. A special case,"
by W. Jadassohn. DERMATOLOGICA. 143:43-44, 1971.

"Choice of penicillins for gonorrhoea." BR MED J. 2:
485, May 29, 1971.

"Chronic monilial vaginitis," by H. Hosen. ANN ALLERGY.
29:499, September, 1971.

"Clinical and epidemiological study of Nicolas-Favre
disease in Bordeaux," by J. M. Tamisier, et al.
BORD MED. 4:739-742 passim, March, 1971.

"Clinical and experimental results in colpitis therapy
using Mysteclin," by H. Lohmeyer, et al. MED KLIN.
66:1278-1280, September 17, 1971.

"Clinical and factorial evaluation of 110 CBFP reacôrs."
by E. A. Johansson. ACTA DERM VENEREOL. 51:Supple-
ment, 65:1-37, 1971.

"Clinical and therapeutic aspects of syphilis," by H.
Storck. PRAXIS. 60:412-419, March 30, 1971.

"Clinical evaluation of carbenoxolone in balanitis,"
by G. W. Csonka, et al. BR J VENER DIS. 47:179-181,
June, 1971.

"Clinical evaluation of the T. pallidum haemagglutination test," by T. Uete, et al. BR J VENER DIS. 47:
73-76, April, 1971

"Clinical, immunochemical and serological studies of
dementia paralytica (GPI)," by H. Schmidt, et al.
INT ARCH ALLERGY APPL IMMUNOL. 40:851-860, 1971.

"Clinical pharmacological aspects of a new hormone derivative (3-tetrahydropyranyl ether of 17-beta-estradiol),"

by C. Andreoli, et al   MINERVA GINECOL.   23:711-724, September 30, 1971.

"Clinical picture of combined gonorrheal-trichomonad urethritis." by I. I. Mavrov, et al.   VESTN DERMATOL VENEROL.   45:84-86, June, 1971.

"Clinical progression of ocular syphilis and neurosyphilis despite treatment with massive doses of penicillin.   Failure to demonstrate treponemes in affected tissues," by C. N. Sowmini.   BR J VENER DIS.   47:348-355, October, 1971.

"Clinical trials with ampicillin in the treatment of gonorrheal urethritis in males," by S. Arap.   HOSPITAL (Rio de Janeiro).   77:1173-1177, April, 1970.

"Clinico-laboratory data on penicillin therapy of patients with gonorrhea," by M. N. Varshavskaya, et al.   VESTN DERMATOL VENEROL.   45:53-56, 1971.

"Clinico-prognostic significance of the Treponema pallidum immobilization reaction in patients with seroresistant syphilis," by IuK Skripkin, et al.   VESTN DERMATOL VENEROL.   45:58-62, January, 1971.

"Clinico-radiologic manifestations of gummatous syphilis involving the soft tissues," by P. D. Khazov.   VESTN DERMATOL VENEROL.   45:85-87, February, 1971.

"The clock is ticking," by M. Strage.   TODAYS HEALTH.   49:16-18 plus, April, 1971

"Clues about carriers; experiments with chimpanzees."   NEWSWEEK.   78:53, July 5, 1971

"A combination of primary syphilis and trichomonal balanoposthitis," by E. L. Fridman.   VESTN DERMATOL VENEROL.   45:67-69, 1971.

"Communities strike back," by W. F. Swartz.   AMER J NURS.   71:724, April, 1971.

"Comparative microscopy, culture and serology studies on Trichomonas vaginalis," by K. J. Beck, et al. GEBURTS-HILFE FRAUENHEILKD. 31:551-560, June, 1971.

"A comparative study of the laboratory diagnosis of gonorrhea," by J. R. Hodges, et al. HEALTH LAB SCI. 8:17-20, January, 1971.

"Comparative study of serologic reactions for the diagnosis of syphilis," by A. Sirena, et al. PRENSA MED ARGENT. 58:1691-1695, October 22, 1971.

"Comparison of direct and indirect fluorescent antibody methods for staining Treponema pallidum," by F. J. Elsas. BR J VENER DIS. 47:255-258, August, 1971.

"Complement-fixing antibodies to Bedsonia in Reiter's syndrome, TRIC agent infection, and control groups," by J. Schachter. AM J OPHTHALMOL. 71:857-860, April, 1971.

"The condom," by K. Flegel. N ENGL J MED. 286:218-219, January 27, 1972.

"Congenital syphilis." ETHIOP MED J. 8:161-162, October, 1970.

"Congenital syphilis," by N. O. Bwibo EAST AFR MED J. 48:185-191, April, 1971.

"Congenital syphilis," by W. H. Eaglstein. ARCH DERMATOL. 103:524-526, May, 1971.

"Congenital syphilis," by T. C. Fleming, et al. J BONE JOINT SURG. 53:1648-1651, December, 1971.

"Congenital syphilis," by Z. Sternadel. PIELEG POLOZNA. 7:10-11, July, 1970.

"Congenital syphilis and its prevention," by D. L. Pereldik. FELDSHER AKUSH. 36:26-29, April, 1971.

"Congenital syphilis in Addis ababa," by Y. Larsson, et al. ETHIOP MED J. 8:163-172, October, 1970.

"Congenital syphilis in the newborn infant: clinical and pathological observations in recent cases," by E. H. Oppenheimer, et al. JOHNS HOPKINS MED J. 129:63-82, August, 1971.

"Congenital syphilis: a nonvenereal disease," by J. G. Caldwell. AM J NURS. 71:1768-1772, September, 1971.

"Congenital syphilis: resurgence of an old problem," by R. H. Wilkinson, et al. PEDIATRICS. 47:27-30, January, 1971.

"Continuous penicillin therapy of patients with infectious syphilis," by M. P. Frishman, et al. VESTN DERMATOL VENEROL. 44:52-57, September, 1970.

"Continuous treatment of early forms of syphilis with penicillin and bicillin," by IuF Korolev. VOEN MED ZH. 7:76-77, 1971.

"Control of venereal diseases." LANCET. 2:807-808, October 9, 1971.

"Control of venereal diseases in Petrograd, 1918-1919," by V. A. Bazanov. VESTN DERMATOL VENEROL. 45:65-69, 1971.

"Cortuitous discovery of a positive syphilitic serology (attempted interpretation and management)," by M. J. Maleville. BORD MED. 4:747-748 passim, March, 1971.

"Corynebacterium vaginale vaginitis in pregnant women," by J. F. Lewis, et al. AM J CLIN PATHOL. 56:580-583, November, 1971.

"Cranial lacunas in secondary syphilis," by P. Amblard, et al. BULL SOC FR DERMATOL SYPHILIGR. 78:310-311, 1971.

"Cranial lacunar osteitis in secondary syphilis," by
G. Cabanel, et al. PRESSE MED. 79:1755-1756, September 25, 1971.

"Cryoglobulin and rheumatoid factor during primosecondary
syphilis," by H. Perrot, et al. PRESSE MED. 7:1059-1060, May 8, 1971.

"Current aspects of blennorrhagia. Statistical study of
200 patients," by P. Amblard, et al. BULL SOC FR DERMATOL SYPHILIGR. 78:188-190, 1971.

"Current aspects of gonococcal disease," by L. Rouques.
PRESSE MED. 7:1077, May 8, 1971.

"Current aspects of gonorrhea. Statistical study apropos
of 200 patients," by P. Amblard, et al. LYON MED. 225-644, April 11, 1971.

"The current course of female gonorrhea," by J. Bartunek.
Z HAUT GESCHLECHTSKR. 46:91-93, February 1, 1971.

"Current epidemiological value of prophylactic serological tests," by J. Lesiński, et al. PRZEGL DERMATOL.
58:163-168, March-April, 1971.

"Current features in current syphilis therapy," by V.
A. Rudaev. FELDSHER AKUSH. 36:26-29, August, 1971.

"Current problems concerning trichomoniasis," by R. Bredland. TIDSSKR NOR LAEGEFOREN. 91:379-381, February
20, 1971.

"The current state of treatment of gonorrhoea with reference to decreased penicillin sensitivity of Neisseria
gonorrhoeae," by J. Meyer-Rohn. BR J VENER DIS. 47:
379, October, 1971.

"The current status of gonorrhoea control," by R. R.
Wilcox. BR J CLIN PRACT. 25:215-222, May, 1971.

"Cutaneous and venereal diseases seen at a drug-oriented

youth clinic," by R. N. Richards. ARCH DERMATOL. 104:438-440, October, 1971.

"Dangers of venereal disease in the family," by S. Chirit-escu. MUNCA SANIT. 19:477-484, August, 1971.

"Decree of Presidium of the Russian Republic supreme soviet no. 881, amending and supplementing the Russian Republic criminal code and criminal procedure code." CURRENT DIG SOVIET PR. 23:24, November 23, 1971.

"Demonstration of the allergic delayed-reaction type in mice following sensitization with Trichomonas vaginalis and a further contribution on the specificity of the peritoneal cell reaction," by R. Michel. Z TROPENMED PARASITOL. 22:91-97, March, 1971.

"Demonstration of the antifungal effect of Candistatin paste, a new nystatin preparation, after storage," by J. O. Toyosi, et al. MYKOSEN. 14:145-147, March 1, 1971.

"Demonstration of the endocytosis process and lysosome structures in Trichomonas vaginalis," by G. Brugerolle C R ACAD SCI. 272:2558-2560, May 17, 1971.

"Demonstration of the inhibitory effect of blood on respiration of Candida albicans using Warburg's apparatus, by J. Kapell, et al. ARCH HYG BAKTERIOL. 154:524-532, April, 1971.

"Demonstration of neisseria gonorrhoeae urethritis," by D. Danielsson, et al. ACTA DERM VENEREOL. 51:73-76, 1971.

"Dermatological and venereal diseases told about in the Bible," by B. Bafverstedt. LAKARTIDNINGEN. 68:3793-3802, August 18, 1971.

"The dermatologist and pruritus ani," by J. E. Racouchot,

et al. AM J PROCTOL. 22:191-195, June, 1971.

"Desoxyribonuclease in Neisseria gonorrhoeae," by U.
Berger. NATURWISSENSCHAFTEN. 58:63, January, 1971.

"Detection of the antitrichomonal drug nitrimidazine
(Naxogin) in urine," by G. D. Morrison, et al. BR J
VENER DIS. 47:38-39, February, 1971.

"Detection of incomplete antibodies in the blood serum
of patients with infectious forms of syphilis and some
dermatoses," by L. S. Reznikova, et al. VESTN DER-
MATOL VENEROL. 45:44-51, August, 1971.

"Detection of Trichomonas vaginalis in patients with
complaints of leukorrhea and the effects of treatment with methylmercadone at the Kurume University,"
by S. Kato, et al. SANFUJINKA JISSAI. 20:884-889,
August, 1971.

"Determination of antibodies against Neisseria gonorrhoeae in gonorrhea patients," by E. Pulchartova, et
al. CESK EPIDEMIOL MIKROBIOL IMUNOL. 20:270-276,
September, 1971.

"Diagnosis and therapy of male urethritis," by J. Meyer-
Rohn. Z HAUT GESCHLECHTSKR. 46:153-158, March 1,
1971.

"Diagnosis and treatment of syphilis," by P. F. Sparling.
N ENGL J MED. 284:642-653, March 25, 1971.

"Diagnosis and treatment of venereal disease," by M. T.
Foster, Jr. POSTGRAD MED. 50:67-73, July, 1971.

"Diagnosis of gonorrhea," by J. Meyer-Rohn. Z ALLGE-
MEINMED. 47:883-886, June 20, 1971.

"Diagnosis of gonorrhea with laboratory-technical methods, including the specific immunofluorescence test
(FAT-Fluorescence Antibody Technic). II. Preparation of immune serums against Neisseria gonorrhoeae

and studies on sensitization and specificity after labelling," by J. Mohr, et al. DTSCH GESUNDHEITSW. 26:1758-1761, September 9, 1971.

"Diagnosis of gonorrheal infection by culture of the external ear canal in the newborn," by J. W. Scanlon. CLIN PEDIATR. 10:528-529, September, 1971.

"The diagnosis of infectious syphilis," by F. B. Desmond. NZ MED J. 73:135-138, March, 1971.

"Diagnosis of Trichomonas foetus infection in bulls," by B. L. Clark, et al. AUST VET J. 47:181-183, May, 1971.

"Diagnostic criteria in candidiasis," by L. Bienias. POL TYG LEK. 26:222-225, July 8, 1971.

"Diagnostic value of the Roemer and Schlipkoeter test in serodiagnosis of late syphilis," by L. Abate, et al. ARCISP S ANNA FERRARA. 23:309-315, 1970.

"Diaper thrush," by W. Gschwandtner, et al. Z HAUT GESCH-LECHTSKR. 46:179-183, March 15, 1971.

"Differential diagnosis of virus hepatitis against hepatic syphilis," by O. Granicki, et al. POL TYG LEK. 26:276-278, February 22, 1971.

"Differing patterns of wheal and flare skin reactivity in patients allergic to the penicillins," by R. G. Van Dellen, et al. J ALLERGY. 47:230-236, April, 1971.

"Direct and delayed methods of immunofluorescent diagnosis of gonorrhoea in women," by R. N. Thin, et al. BR J VENER DIS. 47:27-30, February, 1971.

"Disseminated gonococcal infection," by K. K. Holmes, et al. ANN INTERN MED. 74:979-993, June, 1971.

"Doctor' attention urged by AMA council to problems of

VD." MICH MED. 70:648, July, 1971.

"Doxycycline treatment of nongonococcal urethritis
with special reference to T-strain mycoplasmas,"
by A. Lassus, et al. BR J VENER DIS. 47:126-
130, April, 1971.

"Drug allergy. I." BR MED J. 2:37-40, April 3, 1971.

--II." BR MED J. 2:100-101, April 10, 1971.

"Drug hits VD-related eye disease." AM DRUGGIST. 163:
34, June 28, 1971.

"Dynamics of antibody subsidence in early symptomatic
syphilis treated with penicillin," by L. Kierśnicka-
Itman, et al. PRZEGL DERMATOL. 58:699-707, November-
December, 1971.

"Early congenital bone syphilis: various clinical and
radiological aspects," by A. Fazzi, et al. REV PAUL
MED. 77:73-76, March, 1971.

"Early syphilitic hepatitis. A possible case," by R.
A. Le Clair. BR J VENER DIS. 47:212, June, 1971.

"The economic repercussions of venereal diseases," by
A. E. Callin. BOL OF SANIT PANAM. 70:95-102, January, 1971.

"The effect of antibiotic therapy on mycoplasma in the
female genital tract. In vivo and vivo studies on
the sensitivity of Mycoplasma hominis and T-Mycoplasmas to tetracyclines and other antibiotics," by L.
Weström, et al. ACTA OBSTET GYNECOL SCAND. 50:25-31,
1971.

"Effect of biotin on growth of Candida tropicalis K-41
and synthesis of vitamin B complex," by E. I. Kvasnikov, et al. MIKROBIOL ZH. 33:240-243, March-April,

1971.

"Effect of corticosteroids on the Jarisch-Herxheimer reaction," by A. Luger, et al. WIEN KLIN WOCHEN-SCHR. 83:208-212, March 26, 1971.

"Effect of different immunization procedures on agglutination and precipitation reactions of Trichomonas gallinae," by B. M. Honingsberg, et al. J PARASITOL. 57:363-369, April, 1971.

"Effect of double dose of aqueous procaine penicillin to treat gonorrhea in men," by M. Nelson. HSMHA HEALTH REP. 86:285-288, March, 1971.

"Effect of nystatin on mycelial transformation of Candida albicans cells in the human serum," by H. Buluk, et al. MED DOSW MIKROBIOL. 23:175-181, 1971.

"Effect of penicillin and bicillin-1 in experimental syphilis in rabbits (experimental electron microscopic study," by N. M. Ovchinnikov, et al. VESTN DERMATOL VENEROL. 45:42-47, June, 1971.

"Effect of pyrimidine derivatives on the formation of anti-Candida immunity," by E. N. Bol'shakova. ZH MIKROBIOL EPIDEMIOL IMMUNOBIOL. 48:59-61, February, 1971.

"Effectiveness of condoms in preventing V.D.," by N. J. Fiumara. N ENGL J MED. 285:972, October 21, 1971.

"Effects of the increasing frequency of adult contagious syphilis on those of newborn infants and infants in the Lille and Douai areas since 1962," by F. Desmons. PEDIATRIE. 26:429-432, June, 1971.

"Efficacy of prolonged regimes of oxytetracycline in the treatment of nongonococcal urethritis," by J. John. BR J VENER DIS. 47:266-268, August, 1971.

"Electro-clinical correlations in neurosyphilis," by

C. Postelnicu, et al. ELECTROENCEPHALOGR CLIN NEURO-
PHYSIOL. 30:361, April, 1971.

"Electron microscopic observations on the structure of
Treponema zuelzerae and its axial filiments," by M.
A. Bharier, et al. J BACTERIOL. 105:413-421, Janu-
ary, 1971.

"Electron microscopy of endoflagella and microtubules
in Treponema reiter," by K. H. Hougen, et al. ACTA
PATHOL MICROBIOL SCAND. 79:37-50, 1971.

"Elimination of intercurrent death among rabbits inocu-
lated with Treponema pallidum," by H. J. Jensen. ACTA
PATHOL MICROBIOL SCAND. 79:124-125, 1971.

"Endemic syphilis, venereal syphilis, diseases of the
civilization," by J. Tisseuil. BULL SOC PATHOL EXOT.
64:296-300, May-June, 1971.

"Enzootic typhlitis in the course of mass invasion of
Trichomonas gallinarum in chickens," by S. Stepkow-
ski, et al. WIAD PARAZYTOL. 17:403-410, 1971.

"Enzymatic oxidation of hydrocarbons in Candida inter-
media cells," by L. A. Levchenko, et al. BIOKHIMIIA.
36:88-91, January-February, 1971.

"Epidemic spread." WORLD HEALTH. May, 1971, p. 13.

"Epidemiologic associations between vaginal candidiasis
in the pregnant woman and oral thrush in newborn infants," by A. M. Dolgopol'skaia, et al. VOPR OKHR
MATERIN DET. 16:50-54, February, 1971.

"Epidemiological situation of lues and gonorrhea," by
D. Petzoldt. MED KLIN. 66:335-338, March 5, 1971.

"Epidemiology of gonococci with decreased sensitivity
to penicillin in Malmö, South Sweden," by H. Möller.
ACTA DERM VENEREOL. 51:77-80, 1971.

"Epidemiology of syphilis," by H. Tsugami, et al.
SAISHIN IGAKU. 26:1890-1896, October, 1971.

"Epidemiology of 25,294 reported gonorrhea cases," by
G. R. Najem, et al. J OKLA STATE MED ASSOC. 64:
235-240, June, 1971.

"Epidemy of soft chancres (9 cases)," by H. Thiers, et
al. BULL SOC FR DERMATOL SYPHILIGR. 78:202, 1971.

"Eradication of syphilis," by S. Jonas, et al. N ENGL
J MED. 285:412, August 12, 1971.

"Errors in the diagnosis of acute and chronic nonspecific
epididymitis," by B. S. Gekhman. VOEN MED ZH. 1:43-
45, January, 1971.

"The essential elements of a syphilis control program,"
by W. J. Brown. BOL OF SANIT PANAM. 70:59-65, January, 1971.

"Estimation of dermatophytes (ringworm fungi) and candida spores in the environment," by Y. M. Clayton, et
al. J MED MICROBIOL. 4:p3-P4, May, 1971.

"Evaluation of 'atypical' variants of the results in the
specific syphilis serology," by L. Krell, et al. DTSCH
GESUNDHEITSW. 26:1712-1716, September 2, 1971.

"Evaluation of the autoimmune response in syphilis by
use of a modified Jerne method," by N. I. Tumasheva,
et al. VESTN DERMATOL VENEROL. 45:62-64, November,
1971.

"Evaluation of the automated fluorescent treponema antibody test for syphilis," by H. J. Hornstein, et al.
J LAB CLIN MED. 77:885-890, May, 1971.

"An evaluation of bovine albumin and sodium glutamate
in the lyophilization of Neisseria gonorrhoeae," by
T. L. Klassen. CAN J MED TECHNOL. 33:147-154, August, 1971.

"Evaluation of the gonococcal complement-fixation test," by C. S. Ratnatunga. BR J VENER DIS. 47:279-288, August, 1971.

"Evaluation of a new oral trichomonicid," by J. Delgado Urdapilleta, et al. GINECOL OBSTET MEX. 29:515-519, May, 1971.

"Evaluation of qualitative hemagglutination test for antibodies to Treponema pallidum," by R. A. Le Clair. J INFECT DIS. 123:668-670, June, 1971.

"Evaluation of the results of the leukocyte agglomeration test in syphilis," by IuA Rodin, et al. VESTN DERMATOL VENEROL. 45:64-68, November, 1971.

"Evaluation of treatment of gonorrhea in males with single doses of minocycline," by W. T. Tyson, Jr., et al. J TENN MED ASSOC. 64:773-777, September, 1971.

"Evaluation of the sensitivity of the gonococcus to antibodies. III.," by G. Niel, et al. PATHOL BIOL. 19:53-54, January, 1971.

"Evolution of syphilitic chancres with virulent Treponema pallidum in the rabbit," by N. N. Izzat, et al. BR J VENER DIS. 47:67-72, April, 1971.

"Examination of cerebrospinal fluid," by V. Cagli. POLICLINICO. 78:466-474, June 1, 1971.

"Experience of work of the Chair of Skin and venereal Diseases in aiding public health organizations," by N. A. Torsuev, et al. VESTN DERMATOL VENEROL. 45: 57-60, September, 1971.

"Experience with the diagnosis and treatment of gonorrhea in women," by V. Palous, et al. CESK DERMATOL. 46:256-261, December, 1971.

"Experimental ascending Candida infections in the urinary tract," by M. Hatala, et al. CAS LEK CESK. 110: 553-558, June 11, 1971.

"Experimental cutaneous Candida albicans infection in guinea-pigs," by J. Van Cutsem, et al. SABOURAUDIA. 9:17-20, March, 1971.

"An experimental investigation of farmer's lung. Comparative study of the pulmonary clearance capacity for Aspergillus fumigatus, Candida albicans and Mycropolyspora faeni in guinea pigs," by C. Voisin, et al. REV FR ALLERGOL. 11:129-136, April-June, 1971.

"Experimental pathology of pathogenic fungi. Microscopic detectable pathiological changes in Candida albicans due to pimaricin," by H. Rieth. MYKOSEN. 14:47-48, January 1, 1971.

"Experiments on the influence of metabolites and antimetabolites on the model of Trichomonas vaginalis. I. Experiments with the vitamin-B 2-complex," by C. P. Christow. ZENTRALBL BAKTERIOL. 217:381-402, July, 1971.

"Exploration of delayed cutaneous hypersensitivity to candidine in newborn and young infants," by R. Carron, et al. PEDIATRIE. 26:259-264, April-May, 1971.

"FTA-ABS and VDRL slide test reactivity in a population of nuns," by J. N. Goldman, et al. JAMA. 217: 53-55, July 5, 1971.

"FTA test in neurosyphilis. Immunologic studies with fluorescent antiglobulins fractionated in serum and in cerebrospinal fluid," by S. Sartoris, et al. G ITAL DERMATOL. 46:330-331, July, 1971.

"False positive Wassermann reaction associated with evidence of enterovirus infection," by R. A. Quaife, et al. J CLIN PATHOL. 24:120-121, March, 1971.

"Familial chronic biologic false-positive seroreactions for syphilis. Report of two families, one with three generations affected," by G. H. Kostant. JAMA. 219: 45-48, January, 1972.

"Fatty acid and hydrocarbon hydroxylation in yeast: role of cytochrome P-450 in Candida tropicalis," by J. M. Lebeault, et al. BIOCHEM BIOPHYS RES COMMUN. 42:413-419, February 5, 1971.

"Fetal growth with congenital syphilis: a quantitative study," by R. L. Naeye. AM J CLIN PATHOL. 55:228-231, February, 1971.

"Five-fluorocytosine and urinary candidiasis," by R. R. Davies, et al. BR MED J. 1:577-579, March 13, 1971.

"Five-fluorocytosine in the treatment of cryptococcal and candida mycoses," by R. J. Fass, et al. ANN INTERN MED. 74:535-539, April, 1971.

"Fluorescence method for determination of gonococci in venereologic practice," by H. Medebach. Z HAUT GESCHLECHTSKR. 46:159-162, March 1, 1971.

"Fluorescent treponemal antibody tests on cerebrospinal fluid," by M. F. Garner, et al. BR J VENER DIS. 47: 356-358, October, 1971.

"Focal fungal infections treated by immunological therapy with emphasis on vaginal moniliasis," by H. Hosen. TEX MED. 67:56-58, October, 1971.

"Frenulumplasty: a method for prophylactic treatment in women with recurring urethritis after coitus," by A. Ingelman-Sundberg. NORD MED. 86:988-989, August 19, 1971.

"Further evaluation of the automated fluorescent treponemal antibody test for syphilis," by E. M. Coffey, et al. APPL MICROBIOL. 21:820-822, May, 1971.

"Further studies of the germ-tube test for Candida albicans identification," by C. T. Dolan, et al. AM J CLIN PATHOL. 55:733-734, June, 1971.

"Gaps in venereology." BR MED J. 2:547, June 5, 1971.

"Genital herpes and cervical cancer," by P. Leinikki, et al. DUODECIM. 87:181-183, 1971.

"Genital herpes and cervical cancer," by A. Singer. BR MED J. 1:458, February 20, 1971.

"Genital herpes in two social groups," by W. E. Rawls, et al. AM J OBSTET GYNECOL. 110:682-689, July 1, 1971.

"Genital herpes infection and non-specific urethritis," by S. Jeansson, et al. BR MED J. 3:247, July 24, 1971.

"Genital herpesvirus hominis type 2 infection: an experimental model in cebus monkeys," by A. J. Nahmias, et al. SCIENCE. 171:297-298, January 22, 1971.

"Genital herpesvirus hominis Type 2 infection of monkeys," by W. T. London, et al. OBSTET GYNECOL. 37:501-503 passim, April, 1971.

"A ghost: soft chancre. Apropos of 2 recent cases," by D. Colomb, et al. LYON MED. 225:647-648, April 11, 1971.

"A glutinous rice culture medium for demonstration of chlamydospores of Candida albicans," by S. Sukroongreung. MYCOPATHOL MYCOL APPL. 43:329-335, March 25, 1971.

"Gonococcal arthritis. A survey of 54 cases," by C. L. Cooke, et al. JAMA. 217:204-205, July 12, 1971.

"The gonococcal arthritis-dermatitis syndrome," by K. K.
Holmes, et al. ANN INTERN MED. 75:470-471, September,
1971.

"Gonococcal arthritis in two patients with active lupus
erythematosus. A diagnostic problem," by J. S. Edelen,
et al. ARTHRITIS RHEUM. 14:557-559, September-October, 1971.

"Gonococcal infections in prepubertal children," by V.
F. Burry, et al. MO MED. 68:691-692, September, 1971.

"Gonococcal meningitis," by H. L. Taubin, et al. N ENGL
J MED. 285:504-505, August 26, 1971.

"Gonococcal ophthalmia neonatorum despite treatment with
antibacterial eye-drops," by C. B. Schofield, et al.
BR MED J. 1:257-259, January 30, 1971.

"Gonococcal pharyngitis and arthritis," by F. LaLana, et
al. ANN INTERN MED. 75:649, October, 1971.

"Gonococcal sepsis," by J. Barr, et al. LAKARTIDNINGEN.
68:4255-4260, September 15, 1971.

"Gonococcal sepsis and arthritis." CALIF MED. 114:18-
25, January, 1971.

"Gonococcal tonsillar infections," by A. Bro-Jorgensen,
et al. BR MED J. 4:660-661, December 11, 1971.

"Gonococcal tonsillitis," by Y. Iqbal. BR J VENER DIS.
47:144-145, April, 1971.

"Gonococcal tysonitis without urethritis after prophylactic post-coital urination," by J. A. Burgess. BR J
VENER DIS. 47:40-41, February, 1971.

"Gonococcal vulvovaginitis and possible peritonitis in
prepubertal girls," by V. F. Burry. AM J DIS CHILD.
121:536-537, June, 1971.

"Gonorrhoea," by W. K. Bernfeld. NURS TIMES. 67:382-383, April 1, 1971.

"Gonorrhea," by G. J. Pazin, et al. AM FAM PHYSICIAN. 3:124-137, June, 1971.

"Gonorrhea and gynecological examination during a health survey," by K. Lindholm, et al. LAKARTIDNINGEN. 68:4263-4264, September 15, 1971.

"Gonorrhea and tonsillitis following genito-oral contact," by L. Hellgren. LAKARTIDNINGEN. 68:569-571, February 3, 1971.

"Gonorrhea diagnosis. Laboratory diagnostic point of view," by D. Danielsson. LAKARTIDNINGEN. 68:4242-4250, September 15, 1971.

"Gonorrhea epidemic." NEWSWEEK. 77:54, April 26, 1971.

"Gonorrhea in the adolescent," by R. Sanders. J TENN MED ASSOC. 64:1052-1054, December, 1971.

"Gonorrhea in children," by A. Mark, et al. LAKARTIDNINGEN. 68:4265-4266, September 15, 1971.

"Gonorrhoea in the family," by J. K. Oates. BR MED J. 3:580, September 4, 1971.

"Gonorrhea in a female out-patient-material," by P. A. Märdh, et al. LAKARTIDNINGEN. 68:4261-4262, September 15, 1971.

"Gonorrhea in women," by M. Hart. JAMA. 216:1609-1611, June 7, 1971.

"Gonorrhea in women," by C. S. Nicol. GYNAEKOL RUNDSCH. 10:182-189, 1970.

"Gonorrhea in women: treatment with sulfamethoxazole and trimethoprim," by C. B. Schofield, et al. J INFECT DIS. 124:533-538, December, 1971.

"Gonorrhea masked by acne vulgaris treatment," by T. A. Cortese, Jr. JAMA. 216:330-331, April 12, 1971.

"The gonorrhea problem: action planning," by R. Grubb, et al. LAKARTIDNINGEN. 68:4285-4288, September 15, 1971.

"Gonorrhoea problems," by S. A. Kvorning. UGESKR LAEGER. 133:1249-1252, July 2, 1971.

"Gonorrhea--salpingitis," by V. Falk. LAKARTIDNINGEN. 68:4250-4254, September 15, 1971.

"The gonorrhea situation today," by H. Hansson. LAKARTIDNINGEN. 68:4239-4241, September 15, 1971.

"Gonorrhea today: problems of diagnosis, management, treatment," by R. C. Reznichek, et al. CALIF MED. 115:32-38, August, 1971.

"Gonorrheal conjunctivitis," by R. W. Thatcher, et al. JAMA. 215:1494-1495, March 1, 1971.

"Gonorrheal-trichomonad urethritis in men," by A. I. Lopatin, et al. VESTN DERMATOL VENEROL. 45:53-56, July, 1971

"Good personality breakdown in patients attending venereal diseases clinics," by E. C. de Kite. BR J VENER DIS. 47:135-141, April, 1971.

"Growing menace of V.D.," by M. Walker. TIMES EDUC SUP. 2948:36, November 19, 1971.

"Growth models of cultures with two liquid phases. V. Substrate dissolved in dispersed phase--experimental observation," by A. Prokop, et al. BIOTECHNOL BIOENG. 13:241-256, March, 1971.

"Haemagglutination by the TRIC group of Chlamydia," by

P. F. Elvin-Lewis, et al. J MED MICROBIOL. 4:31-41, February, 1971.

"Haemophilus influenzae infections of the genital tract," by R. J. Farrand. J MED MICROBIOL. 4:357-358, August, 1971.

"Has the nurse any responsibility in the control of venereal disease in the Nigerian community? I." by M. N. Obayan. NIGER NURSE. 2:17-18 passim, July, 1970.

"The health of women," by J. Peel. BR MED J. 3:267-271, July 31, 1971.

"Herpes simplex: diagnosis and management," by A. P. Ulbrich. J AM OSTEOPATH ASSOC. 70:1196-1198, July, 1971.

"Herpes simplex infections on the genitalia," by S. Jeansson, et al. LAKARTIDNINGEN. 68:467-471, January 27, 1971.

"Herpesvirus antibody and carcinoma in situ of the cervix," by L. W. Catalano, Jr., et al. JAMA. 217:447-450, July 26, 1971.

"Hetacillin in single dose in the treatment of gonorrhea," by J. M. de Barros, et al. REV SAUDE PUBLICA. 5:47-50, June, 1971.

"The high price to pay for permissiveness," by B. Keenan. OBSERVER. August 8, 1971, p. 20.

"Historical review of oculogenital disease," by P. Thygeson. AM J OPHTHALMOL. 71:975-985, May, 1971.

"Horny syphilide," by C. N. Sowmini, et al. BR J VENER DIS. 47:213-215, June, 1971.

"Human serum antibodies reacting with endotoxin from Neisseria gonorrhoeae," by J. A. Maeland, et al. BR J VENER DIS. 47:269-272, August, 1971.

"Hutchinson's teeth and early treatment of congenital
    syphilis," by W. K. Bernfeld. BR J VENER DIS. 47:
    54-56, February, 1971.

"Hyaluronidase activity as a factor of vascular permeabil-
    ity in patients with syphilis during treatment," by
    V. V. Kalugin, et al. VESTN DERMATOL VENEROL. 45:
    56-60, October, 1971.

"Identification of Candida isolated from the cutaneous
    candidiasis by the combined use of confirmatory medium
    and slide agglutination with monofactorial antibodies,"
    by T. Nishikawa, et al. MYCOPATHOL MYCOL APPL. 43:
    269-277, March 25, 1971.

"Immediate results of bicillin-5 treatment of patients
    with infectious forms of syphilis," by Sh Khamidov.
    VESTN DERMATOL VENEROL. 45:41-44, August, 1971.

"Immobilization effects of anticell and antiaxial fil-
    ament sera on Treponama zuelzerae," by M. A. Bharier,
    et al   J BACTERIOL. 105:430-437, January, 1971.

"Immunity conditions in treponematoses," by T. Guthe,
    et al. HAUTARZT. 22:329-333, August, 1971.

"Immunoelectrophoresis (I.E.F.) of the cerebrospinal
    fluid of neuroluetics," by M. Pippione, et al.
    G ITAL DERMATOL. 46:323-324, July, 1971.

"Immunoelectrophoretic studies of immunoglobulins
    in early acquired syphilis," by M. Gibowski, et al.
    PRZEGL DERMATOL. 58:708-713, November-December,
    1971.

"Immunofluorescence reaction using fresh blood in syphilis,"
    by T. I. Milonova. VESTN DERMATOL VENEROL. 45:68-73,
    February, 1971.

"Immunofluorescence studies of candida in human reticuloendothelial phagocytes: implications for immunogenesis and pathogenesis of systemic candidiasis," by C. L. Taschdjian, et al. AM J CLIN PATHOL. 56:50-58, July, 1971.

"Immunofluorescent staining for the detection of Treponema pallidum in early syphilitic lesions," by A. E. Wilkinson, et al. BR J VENER DIS. 47:252-254, August, 1971.

"Immunoglobuline in cerebrospinal fluid. Syphilis and IgG," by H. J. Heitmann. DTSCH MED WOCHENSCHR. 96: 966-967, May 28, 1971.

"Immunologic reactions of humans to cephalosporins," by L. D. Petz. POSTGRAD MED J. 47:suppl:64-69, February, 1971.

"Immunological patterns in syphilis including the question of antibodies. With reference to recent experimental studies," by H. Grossmann, et al. HAUTARZT. 21:245-252, June, 1970.

"Immunological reactivity of patients with gonorrhea," by L. D. Butovetskii, et al. VESTN DERMATOL VENEROL. 45:56-59, 1971.

"Immunological studies on treponemal antigens. II. Serological changes and resistance to infection in rabbits immunized with culture supernatant of avirulent Treponema pallidum," by N. N. Izzat, et al. BR J VENER DIS. 47:335-338, October, 1971.

"The importance of cultural identification of Neisseria gonorrhoeae for the diagnosis of problematic clinical cases," by E. Friedrich, et al. DTSCH GESUNDHEITSW. 26:401-404, February 25, 1971.

"Importance of gonococcal cultures and determination of oxidase activity in the diagnosis of gonorrhea," by B. Raszeja-Kotelba, et al. POL TYG LEK. 26:417-419, March 22, 1971.

"Improved tracing of contacts of heterosexual men with gonorrhoea. Relationship of altered female to male ratios," by E. M. Dunlop, et al. BR J VENER DIS. 47: 192-195, June, 1971.

"In vitro antimicrobial activity of 6-(D(-)-amino-p-hydroxy-phenylacetamido) penicillanic acid, a new semisythetic penicillin," by H. C. Neu, et al. ANTIMICROB AGENTS CHEMOTHER. 10:407-410, 1970.

"In vitro sensitivity of mycoplasmas isolated from various animals and sewage to antibiotics and nitrofurans," by M. Ogata, et al. J ANTIBIOT. 24:443-451, July, 1971.

"In vitro studies on the mechanism of penicillin and ampicillin drug reactions," by Z. H. Haddad, et al. INT ARCH ALLERGY APPL IMMUNOL. 41:72-73, 1971.

"In vitro studies with the antimycoticum chlortritylimid-azole," by W. Ritzerfeld, et al. INT Z KLIN PHARMAKOL THER TOXIKOL. 4:204-206, February, 1971.

"In vivo resistance to metronidazole induced on four recently isolated strains of Trichomonas vaginalis," by I. De Carneri, et al. ARZNEIM FORSCH. 21:377-381, March, 1971.

"Incidence of gonorrhoea," by W. F. Felton." BR MED J. 4:683, December 11, 1971.

"The incidence of syphilis in the Bantu: survey of 587 cases from Baragwanath hospital," by M. Dogliotti. S AFR MED J. 45:8-10, January 2, 1971.

"Incidence of Trichomonas vaginalis and of aspecific vaginitis in an apparently healthy female population. Colposcopic and cytological aspects," by B. Cuscianna, et al. MINERVA GINECOL. 23:270-272, March 31, 1971.

"Incidence of Trichomonas vaginalis infection in the female population of Santiago," by H. Schenone, et al. BOL CHIL PARASITOL. 24:159, July-December, 1969.

"The incidence of trichomoniasis and dysuria in pregnant women in Eastern Uganda," by S. L. Lightman, et al. TROP GEOGR MED. 23:113-113, March, 1971.

"Incidence of vaginal trichomoniasis and microbial flora in hysterectomized patients," by J. M. Arizaga Cruz, et al. GINECOL OBSTET MEX. 29:271-274, March, 1971.

"Incomplete agglutinins against Treponema pallidum," by J. Podwińska, et al. BR J VENER DIS. 47:81-86, April, 1971.

"The increase in venereal disease," by L. Cohn. MED J AUST. 1:171-172, January 16, 1971.

"The indirect immunofluorescence in the serologic diagnosis of systemic candidiasis," by R. Negroni, et al. MYCOPATHOL MYCOL APPL. 43:355-359, March 25, 1971.

"Indirect immunofluorescence reaction in the serodiagnosis of candidiasis," by L. Bienias. MYKOSEN. 14: 115-118, March 1, 1971.

"Infantile congenital syphilis. Presenting with bilateral orchitis," by R. Singh, et al. BR J VENER DIS. 47: 206-208, June, 1971.

"Infection of the urinary system with Trichomonas vaginalis in newborn female infants," by Z. Worwag. WIAD PARAZYTOL. 17:355-358, 1971.

"Influence of gestogenic contraceptive pills on vaginal candidosis," by R. D. Catterall. BR J VENER DIS. 47: 45-47, February, 1971.

"Influence of oral contraception upon the occurence of Candida albicans in the vagina," by H. Thulin. NORD MED. 85:399-401, April 1, 1971.

"The influence of penicillinase on hapten inhibitions in vitro and in vivo in experimental penicillin allergy," by D. Kraft, et al. Z IMMUNITAETSFORSCH ALLERG KLIN IMMUNOL. 141:265-273, 1971.

"Inhibitions with haptens in penicillin allergy," by H. P. Werner, et al. WIEN KLIN WOCHENSCHR. 83:194-196, March 19, 1971.

"Interactions of antilipoidal antibodies with yolk sac antigens," by A. Lassus, et al. BR J VENER DIS. 47: 169-172, June, 1971.

"The international incidence of venereal disease," by T. Guthe, et al. R SOC HEALTH J. 91:122-133, May-June, 1971.

"Intertriginous and genital Candida mycoses," by W. Mein-hof. DTSCH MED WOCHENSCHR. 96:887, May 14, 1971.

"Intrauterine pregnancy and coexistent pelvic inflammatory disease," by A. A. Acosta, et al. OBSTET GYNECOL. 37:282-285, February, 1971.

"Intravascular coagulation and acute renal failure in a child with mycoplasma infection," by I. M. Nilsson, et al. ACTA MED SCAND. 189:359-365, May, 1971.

"Investigations on cultivation and biology of Trichomonas vaginalis," by P. Christoe. ZENTRALB BAKTERIOL. 217:540-553, August, 1971.

"Inveterate explosion fracture dislocation of the neuro-pathic shoulder joint," by O. C. Kestler. BULL HOSP JOINT DIS. 32:63-72, April, 1971.

"Is the pill to blame for V.D. rise?" AM DRUGGIST. 163: 38 plus, May 17, 1971.

"Isolated affection of paraurethral ducts by gonorrheal infection," by F. V. Potapnev, et al. VESTN DERMATOL VENEROL. 45:83-84, June, 1971.

"Isolation of human genital TRIC agents in nongonococcal
urethritis and Reiter's disease by an irradiated cell
culture method," by D. K. Ford, et al. BR J VENER DIS.
47:196-197, June, 1971.

"Isolation of L-form bacteria and mycoplasma in inflammatory urologic diseases," by A. E. Sukhodol'skaia, et
al. VRACH DELO. June, 1971, p. 12-15.

"The isolation of Trichomonads from pigeons," by T. M.
Grimes, et al. AUST VET J. 47:160-161, April, 1971.

"Isovitalex--a chemically definable enricher of culture
media for Neisseria gonorrhoeae," by L. Pospisil.
CESK DERMATOL. 46:23-25, February, 1971.

"Juvenile progressive paralysis," by V. Satková, et al.
CESK PEDIATR. 26:500-501, October, 1971.

"Keratodermia blenorrhagica in Reiter's disease," by R.
Howell. BR MED J. 1:725-726, March 27, 1971.

"A laboratory test is not a diagnosis," by N. J. Fiumara.
JAMA. 217:71, July 5, 1971.

"Langerhans' cells in late pinta. Ultrastructural observations in one case," by H. A. Rodriguez, et al. ARCH
PATHOL. 91:302-306, April, 1971.

"Late results of a complex study of children born to
syphilitic mothers properly treated before and during
pregnancy," by P. E. Pochkhua. VESTN DERMATOL VENEROL.
45:66-67, February, 1971.

"Late results of treating syphilis with bicillin-1,3,4
and bicillin-3,4, in combination with pyrogenal," by

T. V. Vasil'ev. VESTN DERMATOL VENEROL. 45:50-58, January, 1971.

"'Let's get V.D.'" by C. B. Kanterman. DENT STUD. 49: 20, May, 1971

"Life cycle of urogenital trichomonas under the influence of some chemicals," by I. K. Padchenko. PEDIATR AKUSH GINEKOL. 2:53-55, 1971.

"Linear calcification of the aorta," by M. C. Thorner. JAMA. 215:297, January 11, 1971.

"Lipid metabolism in the parasitic and free-living spirochetes Treponema pallidum (Reiter) and Treponema zuelzerae," by H. Meyer, et al. BIOCHIM BIOPHYS ACTA. 231:93-106, February 2, 1971.

"Liver disease associated with early syphilis," by A. L. Baker, et al. N ENGL J MED. 284:1422-1423, June 24, 1971.

"Liver disease associated with secondary syphilis," by R. V. Lee, et al. N ENGL J MED. 284:1423-1425, June 24, 1971.

"The liver in secondary (early) syphilis," by S. Sherlock. N ENGL J MED. 284:1437-1438, June 24, 1971.

"Living environment of Pakistani immigrants attending venereal disease clinics in Britain," by A. S. Hossain. PUBLIC HEALTH. 85:123-131, March, 1971.

"Local treatment of female urethritis," by S. Nilsson. LAKARTIDNINGEN. 68:581-584, February 3, 1971.

"Luetic aneurysm of the descended aortic arch with neurologic complications (case report)," by Z. Novak, et al. NEUROPSIHIJATRIJA. 18:179-189, 1970.

"Luetic thoraco-lumbal aortic aneurysm with arrosion of

the vertebral body," by I. Boldt, et al. FORTSCHR GEB ROENTGENSTR NUKLEARMED. 114:846-849, June, 1971.

"The luminescent method of detecting pupillary disorders in early forms of syphilis," by V. D. Kochetkov, et al. ZH NEVROPATHOL PSIKHIATR. 71:202-204, 1971.

"Lymecycline in Haemophilus vaginalis colpitis," by H. Fegerl, et al. WIEN MED WOCHENSCHR. 121:194-196, March 13, 1971.

"Lymphadenopathy in secondary syphilis," by D. R. Turner. J PATHOL. 104:x, July, 1971.

"Lymphoblastic transformation test during syphilis," by C. Janot, et al. PRESSE MED. 79:1901-1904, October 16, 1971.

"A lyophilization medium for FTA-ABS test antigen," by E. F. Hunter, et al. HEALTH LAB SCI. 8:35-39, January, 1971.

"The maltose metabolism of Trichomonas gallinae (Rivolta, 1878). II. Metabolic studies," by J. J. Daly. J PARASITOL. 57:370-374, April, 1971.

"Management of nonspecific urethritis." BR MED J. 3: 62, July 10, 1971.

"Management of pregnancy complicated by genital herpes virus infection," by M. S. Amstey. OBSTET GYNECOL. 37:515-520, April, 1971.

"Management of sexually assaulted females," by J. B. Massey, et al. OBSTET GYNECOL. 38:29-36, July, 1971.

"Masking of syphilis." BR MED J. 3:206, July 24, 1971.

"Mating responses in Candida lipolytica," by A. I. Herman.   J BACTERIOL.   107:371, July, 1971.

"Mechanism of uptake of liquid hydrocarbons by microorganisms," by F. Yoshida, et al.   BIOTECHNOL BIO-
ENG.   13:215-228, March, 1971.

"Medical inspection of prostitutes in America in the
nineteenth century: the St. Louis experiment and
its sequel," by J. C. Burnham.   BULL HIST MED.   45:
203-218, May-June, 1971.

"A medium for the diagnosis of vaginal Candidiasis,"
by H. Becker, et al.   MYKOSEN.   14:127-130, March
1, 1971.

"Meet the V.D. epidemiologist," by D. C. Vandermeer.
AM J NURS.   71:722-723, April, 1971.

"Meningococci in vaginitis," by J. E. Gregory, et al.
AM J DIS CHILD.   121:423, May, 1971.

"Meningococcus and gonococcus: never the Twain--well,
hardly ever," by H. A. Feldman.   N ENGL J MED.   285:
518-520, August 26, 1971.

"Methionine biosynthesis in Candida albicans.   I.   S-
adenosyl-L-methionine (or S-methyl-L-methionine):
homocysteine methyltransferase in cell-free extracts from yeast-like cells," by D. N. Mardon, et
al.   CAN J MICROBIOL.   17:795-802, June, 1971.

"Metronidazole as a possible reason for difficulty in
diagnosis of syphilis," by I. I. Il'in, et al.
VESTN DERMATOL VENEROL.   45:74-76, February, 1971.

"Microangiopathic hemolysis and thrombocytopenia related to penicillin drugs," by J. C. Parker, et
al.   ARCH INTERN MED.   127:474-477, March, 1971.

"Microbiological study of copiamycin," by K. Seiga, et
al.   APPL MICROBIOL.   21:986-989, June, 1971.

"Microflocculation assay for gonococcal antibody," by G. Reising. APPL MICROBIOL. 21:852-853, May, 1971.

"Microreaction on glass with fresh blood, plasma and active serum in syphilis," by T. I. Milonova, et al. VESTN DERMATOL VENEROL. 45:40-44, May, 1971.

"Microscopy in the diagnosis of gonorrhea," by O. I. Haavelsrud, et al. TIDSSKR NOR LAEGEFOREN. 91:1476-1477, July 10, 1971.

"'Microtiter' technic for VDRL," by S. S. Kasatiya, et al. CAN J PUBLIC HEALTH. 62:61-62, January-February, 1971.

"Modern serology of syphilis. I. Preparation and testing of the cardiolipin antigen for the complement fixation reaction, introduced in production at the 'Dr. I. Cantacuzino Institute'," by M. Georgescu, et al. MICROBIOL PARAZITOL EPIDEMIOL. 16:67-72, January-February, 1971.

"Modern serology of syphilis. II. Preparation for production of a cardiolipin antigen of the VDRL type for serodiagnosis of syphilis with a flocculation reaction. Value and methods of use," by M. Georgescu, et al. MICROBIOL PARAZITOL EPIDEMIOL. 16:263-272, May-June, 1971.

"Modification of the composition and structure of the yeast cell wall by culture in the presence of sulfur amino acids," by K. A. Killick. J BACTERIOL. 106: 931-937, June, 1971.

"Monomycin in treating gonorrhea in women," by E. N. Turanova, et al. VESTN DERMATOL VENEROL. 45:59-62, 1971.

"Morphologic and histochemical changes in the mucosa of the urogenital tract in gonorrhea, trichomonas and candidiasis," by V. G. Bilik, et al. VESTN DERMATOL VENEROL. 45:50-53, May, 1971.

"Mpilo Hospital Round. Euthyroidism, exophthalmos,
acropachy and pretibial myxoedema," by J. E. Thomas.
CENT AFR J MED. 17:23-24, January, 1971.

"Mycoplasma and vaginal cytology," by P. A. Mardh, et
al. ACTA CYTOL. 15:310-315, May-June, 1971.

"Mycplasma hominis and postpartum febrile complications,
by H. J. Harwick, et al. OBSTET GYNECOL. 37:765-
768, May, 1971.

"Mycoplasma pneumoniae pneumonia in Helsinki 1962-1970.
Epidemic pattern and autoimmune manifestations," by
E. Jansson, et al. SCAND J INFECT DIS. 3:51-54, 1971.

"Mycoplasmas and the evidence for their pathogenicity in
man," by D. Taylor-Robinson. PROC R SOC MED. 64:31-
33, January, 1971.

"Mycoplasmas and fertility." DTSCH MED WOCHENSCHR. 96:
223, January 29, 1971.

"A nationwide serum survey of Argentinian military recruits, 1965-1966. I. Description of sample and
antibody patterns with arboviruses, polioviruses,
respiratory viruses, tetanus and treponematosis," by
A. S. Evans, et al. AM J EPIDEMIOL. 93:111-121,
February, 1971.

"Neisseria gonorrhoeae. II. Colony variation," by A.
Reyn, et al. ACTA PATHOL MICROBIOL SCAND. 79:
435-436, 1971.

--III. Demonstration of presumed appendages to cells
from different colony types," by A. E. Jephcott, et
al. ACTA PATHOL MICROBIOL SCAND. 79:437-439, 1971.

"Neisseria gonorrhoeae in prostatic fluid after treatment of uncomplicated gonorrheal urethritis," ACTA
DERM VENEROL. 51:73-76, 1971.

"The Nelson-Mayer TPI-test and the treatment of syphilis in medical practice," by K. Hübschmann. WIEN KLIN WOCHENSCHR. 82:371-373, May 15, 1971.

"Neonatal congenital syphilis. Diagnosis by the anti IgM treponemal fluorescence test," by J. Kipnis, et al. REV INST MED TROP SAO PAULO. 13:179-183, May-June, 1971.

"Nephropathy of secondary syphilis. A clinical and pathological spectrum," by M. S. Bhorade, et al. JAMA. 216:1159-1166, May 17, 1971.

"Nephrotic syndrome: a complication of secondary syphilis by M. D. Hellier, et al. BR MED J. 4:404-405, November 13, 1971.

"Neuro-ophthalmological study of late yaws. I. An intro duction to yaws," by J. L. Smith. BR J VENER DIS. 47:223-225, August, 1971.

--and pinta. II. The Caracas project," by J. L. Smith, et al. BR J VENER DIS. 47:226-251, August, 1971.

"New Arizona legislation for treatment of minors with V.D.," by S. Dandoy. ARIZ MED. 28:529-530, July, 1971.

"New data on the spore tubule formation of Candida albicans in various human and animal serums," by J. O. Toyosi, et al. MYKOSEN. 14:49-51, January 1, 1971.

"New legislation for treating minors with venereal disease," by S. Dandoy. ARIZ NURSE. 24:55, September-October, 1971.

"New method of staining Trichomonas," by P. Francechini. PRESSE MED. 79:486-487, February 27, 1971.

"A new treatment fot monilial vaginitis." PRACTITIONER. 207:236-238, August, 1971.

"Nifuratrone and gonorrhea," by E. B. Smith, et al.
ANTIMICROB AGENTS CHEMOTHER. 10:267-269, 1970.

"Nitrimidazine in the treatment of Trichomonas vaginalis
vaginitis," by L. Cohen. BR J VENER DIS. 47:177-178,
June, 1971.

"Nitrimidazine in the treatment of trichomoniasis," by
M. Moffett, et al. BR J VENER DIS. 47:173-176, June,
1971.

"Nonvenereal transmission of gonococcal infections to
children," by W. B. Shore, et al. J PEDIATR. 79:
661-663, October, 1971.

"A note on congenital abnormalities of the penis. Incidence and relationship to urethritis," by A. I. Morrison.
BR J VENER DIS. 47:182-183, June, 1971.

"The nurse and V.D. control," by H. E. Ferrari. CAN NURSE.
67:28-30, July, 1971.

"Occurrence of fetal syphilis after a nonreactive early
gestational serologic test," by F. L. al-Salihi, et
al. J PEDIATR. 78:121-123, January, 1971.

"Occurrence of latent forms of syphilis in the absence
of manifestations in the beginning stages," by S. I.
Berlin, et al. VESTN DERMATOL VENEROL. 45:45-50,
May, 1971.

"The occurrence of oxidase-positive non-gonococcal
strains on Thayer-Martin selective media used in the
laboratory diagnostic of N. gonorrhoeae," by E. Geizer. ZENTRALBL BAKTERIOL. 214:75-78, 1970.

"Occurrence of Trichomonas vaginalis in the urinary
system of newborn male infants," by Z. Worwag.
WIAD PARAZYTOL. 17:351-354, 1971.

"Occurrence of two maximum temperatures for growth in yeasts," by A. Oliveira-Baptista, et al.   Z ALLG MIKROBIOL.   11:59-61, 1971.

"Ominous follow-up to syphilis."   MED WORLD MEWS.   12:16-17, January 29, 1971.

"On the antibiotic sensitivity of strains of Neisseria gonorrhoeae," by M. Péter, et al.   MICROBIOL PARAZITOL EPIDEMIOL.   16:153-157, March-April, 1971.

"On the etiology of epididymitis," by L. H. Wolin.   J UROL.   105:531-533, April, 1971.

"On the ultrastructure of Trichomonas vaginalis," by D. Panaitescu, et al.   ARCH ROUM PATHOL EXP MICROBIOL.   30:87-106, March, 1971.

"One-capsule treatment of gonorrhea with minocycline," by H. Pariser, et al.   ANTIMICROB AGENTS CHEMOTHER.   10:211-213, 1970.

"One-day oral ampicillin-treatment of gonorrhea in young adults," by L. H. Shapiro, et al.   OBSTET GYNECOL.   37:414-418, March, 1971.

"One of the causes of nonspecific false positive reactions in syphilis," by L. G. Sagdeeva.   VESTN DERMATOL VENEROL.   44:59-64, September, 1970.

"Oral ampicillin in uncomplicated gonorrhoea.   III.   Results of treatment in women with positive rectal culture," by G. Eriksson.   ACTA DERM VENEREOL.   51:305-310, 1971.

"Oral ampicillin in uncomplicated gonorrhoea.   IV.   Comparison of pharmacological and clinical results," by G. Eriksson.   ACTA DERM VENEREOL.   51:467-475, 1971.

"Oral single-dose treatment of male and female gonorrhea with ampicillin alone and combined with probenecid," by A. Bro-Jorgensen, et al.   UGESKR LAEGER.   133:1253-1256, July 2, 1971.

"Osseous yaws and goundou," by L. Cornet, et al. J
    CHIR. 102:101-104, July-August, 1971.

"Other people's disease." EMERGENCY MED. 3:126-127,
    March, 1971.

"Other sexually transmitted diseases. I." by C. S.
    Nicol. BR MED J. 2:448-449, May 22, 1971.

--II." by C. S. Nicol. BR MED J. 2:507-509, May 29,
    1971.

"Overcoming teacher reluctancy toward V.D. education,"
    by F. B. Benell. J SCH HEALTH. 40:483-486, November,
    1970.

"Oxytetracycline-nystatin in the prevention of candidal
    vaginitis," by M. Silverman, et al. AM J OBSTET
    GYNECOL. 111:398-404, October 1, 1971.

"PAM plus probenecid and procaine penicillin plus pro-
    benecid in gonorrhoea," by A. L. Hilton. BR J VENER
    DIS. 47:107-110, April, 1971.

"Paraplegia: An aetiological survey," by A. Singh, et
    al. J INDIAN MED ASSOC. 56:219-223, April 16, 1971.

"Parasitic protozoa in the human oral cavity and their
    clinical importance," by F. A. Musaev. STOMATOLOGIIA.
    50:60-62, May-June, 1971.

"Partial epidemiological analysis of gonorrhea cases in
    a single Prague district," by K. Kopecký, et al. CESK
    EPIDEMIOL MIKROBIOL IMMUNOL. 20:195-202, July, 1971.

"Participation of the Department of Dermatologic and
    Venereal Diseases of the Grodno Medical Institute in
    the work of regional dermato-venereological network,"
    by L. I. Gokinaeva. VESTN DERMATOL VENEROL. 45:60-61,
    June, 1971.

"Pathogenesis and treatment of seroresistant syphilis," by A. A. Studnitsin, et al. VESTN DERMATOL VENEROL. 45:47-52, June, 1971.

"Pathogenesis of pupillary disorders in various forms of syphilis of the nervous system," by V. D. Kochetkov, et al. VESTN DERMATOL VENEROL. 44:53-58, March, 1970

"Pathogenetic value of intracranial blood flow in a case of median cerebral artery occlusion associated with homolateral hemiplegia," by J. Solé-Llenas, et al. NEUROCHIRURGIA. 14:225-231, November, 1971.

"Penicillin 'fatigue'," by K. Naess. TIDSSKR NOR LAE-GEFOREN. 91:665-666, March 30, 1971.

"Penicillin therapy in 44 cases of primary and secondary syphilis," by B. A. Smithurst. MED J AUST. 2:248-250 July 31, 1971.

"Perinatal risk associated with maternal genital herpes," by A. J. Nahmias, et al. AM J OBSTET GYNECOL. 110: 825-837, July 15, 1971.

"Perinatal tips," by P. M. Zavell. MICH MED. 70:123-124, February, 1971.

"Persistence of T. pallidum and its significance in penicillin-treated seropositive late syphilis," by L. Yogeswari, et al. BR J VENER DIS. 47:339-347, October, 1971.

"Perspectives in the treatment of protozoal diseases resistant to metronidazole," by I. De Carneri. TRANS R SOC TROP MED HYG. 65:268-270, 1971.

"A phenomenon resembling opsonic adherence shown by dis-aggregated cells of the tranmissible venereal tumour of the dog," by D. Cohen, et al. BR J EXP PA-THOL. 52:447-451, October, 1971.

"Physiologic changes during the Jarisch-Herxheimer reaction in early syphilis. A comparison with louse-borne relapsing fever," by D. A. Warrell, et al. AM J MED. 51:176-185, August, 1971.

"Pimafucin--a polyvalent vaginal therapeutic agent," by U. Heynen. Z ALLGEMEINMED. 47:829-830, June 31, 1971.

"Polyester sponge swabs to facilitate examination for genital infection in women," by J. K. Oates, et al. BR J VENER DIS. 47:289-292, August, 1971.

"Polyneuritis in the course of early latent syphilis," by K. Hulanicka, et al. NEUROL NEUROCHIR POL. 5: 121-124, 1971.

"Positive fluorescent treponemal antibody test in systemic lupus erythematosus in childhood: report of a case," by R. P. Lesser, et al. J PEDIATR. 79: 1006-1008, December, 1971.

"Possibilities in influencing the occurrence of trichomoniasis," by M. Valent. BRATISL LEK LISTY. 56: 21-28, 1971.

"Possibility of the transmission of syphilis in the blood of a donor with a latent form of this disease," by A. A. Mikhailova, et al. PROBL GEMATOL PERELIV KROVI. 16:50-51, July, 1971.

"Postirradiation vaginitis. An evaluation of prophylaxis with topical estrogen," by R. M. Pitkin, et al. RADIOLOGY. 99:417-421, May, 1971.

"Practical evaluation of culture media with SCA basis produced by the Serology and Vaccine Institute," by V. Resl, Jr., et al. CESK DERMATOL. 46:29-38, February, 1971.

"Practical interpretation of serologic tests for syphilis," by M. Renoux. PRESSE MED. 79:685-

689, March 24, 1971.

"A preliminary study of the treponemal pallidum haemagglutination test (TPHA)," by S. Vejjajiva, et al. J MED ASSOC THAI. 54:256-259, April, 1971.

"Present pattern of antibiotic sensitivity of gonococcal strains isolated in Bombay," by J. M. Moses, et al. BR J VENER DIS. 47:273-278, August, 1971.

"Present trends in the laboratory diagnosis of N. gonorrhoeae," by R. M. Breen. MED ANN DC. 40:638-639, October, 1971.

"The preservation of gonococci in liquid nitrogen," by M. E. Ward, et al. J CLIN PATHOL. 24:122-123, March, 1971.

"Prevention of communicable diseases in Mexico. V. Pinta. Situation in Mexico in 1970," by G. Gosset-Osuna. GAC MED MEX. 101:167-175, February, 1971.

"Prevention of vaginal Candida proliferation by the use of Pimafucin vaginal tablets during metronidazole treatment," by I. Alteras. BRUX MED. 51:501-503, July, 1971.

"The prevention of venereal disease," by V. G. Cave. J NATL MED ASSOC. January, 1971, p. 66-68.

"Primary gonorrheal abscess of the penile skin," by Z. Ruszczak, et al. PRZEGL DERMATOL. 58:627-629, September-October, 1971.

"Principle and effect of anti-treponema pallida specific syphilis tests FTA and TPI," by G. Blaurock, et al. DTSCH GESUNDHEITSW. 26:1152-1156, June 17, 1971.

"Problem of latent syphilis," by L. A. Rozina, et al. VESTN DERMATOL VENEROL. 45:57-59, June, 1971.

"The problem of penicillin allergy," by J. W. Smith. ARIZ MED. 28:305-307, April, 1971.

"The problem of venereal diseases in the Americas," by A. Llopis. BOL OF SANIT PANAM. 70:26-58, January, 1971.

"The problem of venereal diseases in Singapore," by R. S. Morton. BR J VENER DIS. 47:48-51, February, 1971.

"Problems in the control of blenorrhagia," by A. Campos Salas. BOL OF SANIT PANAM. 70:66-78, January, 1971.

"Problems in social medicine," by V. H. Wallace. MED J AUST. 2:828-829, October 16, 1971.

"Progonasyl for V.D. prophylaxis?" by E. H. Braff. CALIF MED. 115:75, October, 1971.

"Progressive sypilitic paresis in a 12-year-old girl," by Z. Goscinska, et al. PEDIATR POL. 46:369-371, March, 1971.

"Prophylactic treatment with penicillin in venereal diseases," by A. Luger. HAUTARZT. 22:135, March, 1971.

"Prophylaxis of gonococcal ophthalmia." MED LETT DRUGS THER. 12:38-39, May 1, 1970.

"The prostate as a reservoir for gonococci," by D. Danielsson, et al. LAKARTIDNINGEN. 68:4267 passim, September 15, 1971.

"Proteinogram and results of immunofluorescence tests in the examination of dried sera of patients with syphilis," by S. M. Vorobeichik, et al. VESTN DERMATOL VENEROL. 45:45-50, October, 1971.

"Pruritus vulvae," by C. N. Hudson. BR MED J. 1:656-657, March 20, 1971.

"Psychological aspects in venereology," by F. Novotny.
CESK DERMATOL. 46:77-82, April, 1971.

"Psychopathology in V.D. practice," by A. N. Boneff.
INDIAN J DERMATOL. 16:51-54, April, 1971.

"Psycho-social aspects of venereal diseases in teen-
agers," by I. Datt. INDIAN J DERMATOL. 16:27-35,
January, 1971.

"The public health investigator's expanding role," by
T. W. Mathias, et al. HSMHA HEALTH REP. 86:107-110,
February, 1971.

"Public health report." CALIF MED. 115:78-79, October,
1971.

"Pyrolysis-gas chromatography of polyene antifungal antibiotics: The nature of candicidin, levorin and trichomycin," by H. J. Burrows, et al. J CHROMATOGR. 53:
566-571, December 23, 1971.

Quantitative determination and serological activity of
19S- and 7S-immunoglobulins in syphilis II," by E.
Kuwert, et al. Z IMMUNITAEFORSCH EXP KLIN IMMUNOL.
141:303-316, April, 1971.

"Quantitative study of immunoglobulins in the cerebrospinal fluid of neuroluetics," by G. Martina, et al.
G ITAL DERMATOL. 46:322-323, July, 1971.

"Rapid identification of yeasts of the Candida albicans
and Candida tropicalis specific by slide agglutination with species serum," by M. Sefer, et al. ROM
MED REV. 15:8-10, January-March, 1971.

"Rapid plasma diagnosis of syphilis," by G. Nicolau,
et al. ROM MED REV. 15:44-48, January-March, 1971.

"Rapid plasma reagin (RPR) card test. A screening method for treponemal disease," by A. N. Walker. BR J VENER DIS. 47:259-262, August, 1971.

"Rare cases of Herxheimer's reaction in a 1-month-old infant with hemolytic jaundice in the course of congenital syphilis," by K. Jaegermann. PRZEGL EPIDEMIOL. 25:441-443, 1971.

"The reaction of the isoenzymes of transaldolase with chlorodinitrobenzene," by O. Tsolas, et al. ARCH BIOCHEM BIOPHYS. 143:516-525, April, 1971.

"Reappearance of soft chancre (5 cases)," by H. Perrot, et al. BULL SOC FR DERMATOL SYPHILIGR. 78:200-201, 1971; also in: LYON MED. 225:649-650, April 11, 1971.

"Re-appraising the effect on incubating syphilis of treatment for gonorrhoea," by K. R. Woodcock. BR J VENER DIS. 47:95-101, April, 1971.

"Recommendations on the diagnosis of gonorrhea," by A. H. Rudolph, et al. JAMA. 218:448, October 18, 1971.

"Record of a case of gonorrhea." INFIRM FR. 123:33, March, 1971.

"Recovery of Neisseria gonorrhoeae from 'Sterile' synovial fluid in gonococcal arthritis," by K. K. Holmes, et al. N ENGL J MED. 284:318-320, February 11, 1971.

"Rectal gonorrhea in women," by K. Odegaard, et al. TIDSSKR NOR LAEGEFOREN. 91:1474-1476, July 10, 1971.

"Recurrence of soft chancre. 2 recent cases," by D. Colomb, et al. BULL SOC FR DERMATOL SYPHILIGR. 78:197-199, 1971.

"Reduced maternal plasma and urinary estriol during

ampicillin treatment," by K. Willman, et al. AM
J OBSTET GYNECOL. 109:893-896, March 15, 1971.

"Reiter's disease," by J. J. De Blecourt. NED TIJD-
SCHR GENEESKD. 115:97-100, January 16, 1971.

"Relationship of herpes simplex genital infection and
carcinoma of the cervix: population studies," by
Y. M. Centifanto, et al. AM J OBSTET GYNECOL. 110:
690-692, July 1, 1971.

"Relationship of Torulopsis to candida," by B. G.
Leask, et al. LANCET. 1:1300-1301, June 19, 1971.

"Repeated syphilis infection after treatment by a
permanent method," by M. Z. Kagan, et al. VESTN
DERMATOL VENEROL. 45:76-79, September, 1971.

"The reporting of venereal diseases by physicians,"
by R. H. Vanderhook. J INDIANA STATE MED ASSOC.
64:1187-1188, November, 1971.

"Reports from the obstetrical clinic in Leipzig. Prevention of eye inflamation in the newborn." AM J
DIS CHILD. 121:3-4, January, 1971.

"Research on the treponematoses." WHO CHRON. 25:112-
116, March, 1971.

"Resistance and serological changes in rabbits immunized with virulent Treponema pallidum sonicate,"
by N. N. Izzat, et al. ACTA DERM VENEROL. 51:157-
160, 1971.

"Responsibility of the physician in the control of
venereal disease." NY STATE J MED. 71:1717,
July 15, 1971.

"Results of electroencephalography in early and latent syphilis," by N. V. Bratus' et al. VESTN
DERMATOL VENEROL. 45:50-53, July, 1971.

"Results of the Nelson test during administration of gentamycin," by H. J. Heitmann, et al. Z HAUT GESCHLECHTSKR. 46:87-90, February 1, 1971.

"Results of treatment of gonorrhea with penicillin in the light of clinical observations and laboratory examinations," by J. Bowszyc, et al. PRZEGL DERMATOL. 58:715-721, November-December, 1971.

"Results of treatment with trimethoprim-sulfamethoxazole in dermovenereology," by S. D. Randazzo. G ITAL DERMATOL. 46:269-272, June, 1971.

"Resurgence of gonorrhea and its diagnosis by the gono-reaction," by E. Russo. REV BRAS MED. 28:99-103, March, 1971.

"Return to nursing: Changes in dermatology," by N. Thorne. NURS MIRROR. 133:30-35, September 3, 1971.

"Review of hospitalized cases of general paralysis of the insane," by K. Dawson-Butterworth, et al. BR J VENER DIS. 46:295-302, August, 1970.

"A review of 'Microbes and morals' by T. Rosebury," by A. Cooper. NEWSWEEK. 78:95B-96, October 4, 1971.

"Rifadin (rifampicin) in treatment of gonorrhoea in Uganda. A controlled trial," by O. P. Arya, et al. BR J VENER DIS. 47:184-187, June, 1971.

"Role of mycoplasma infection in the genesis of spontaneous abortion," by M. A. Bashmakova, et al. VOPR OKHR MATERIN DET. 16:67-70, February, 1971.

"The role of sorbent in the absorbed fluorescent treponamal antibody (FTA-ABS) test," by A. E. Wilkinson, et al. PROC R SOC MED. 64:422-425, April, 1971.

"Routine use of penicillin skin testing on an inpatient service," by N. F. Adkinson, Jr.   N ENGL J MED.   285:22-24, July 1, 1971.

"The St. Claire County gonorrhea study: Private and public health resources combine in an effort to control gonorrhea," by R. E. Rowe, et al.   MICH MED.   70:317-318, April, 1971.

"Salivary vulvitis," by B. A. Davis.   OBSTET GYNECOL. 37:238-240, February, 1971.

"Sarcoid-like granulomas in secondary syphilis.   A clinical and histopathologic study of five cases," by L. B. Kahn, et al.   ARCH PATHOL.   92:334-337, November, 1971.

"Sarcoidal reaction of the skin in syphilis," by R. Singh, et al.   BR J VENER DIS.   47:209-211, June, 1971.

"Scanning electron microscopic studies of Candida albicans," by W. G. Barnes, et al.   J BACTERIOL.   106: 276-280, April, 1971.

"Schizophrenic syndrome in congenital syphilis," by O. Skalicková, et al.   CESK PSYCHIATR.   67:260-264, October, 1971.

"Screening females for asymptomatic gonorrhea infection," by A. H. Pedersen, et al.   NORTHWEST MED. 70:255-261, April, 1971.

"Screening tests for gonorrhea in clinics for contraceptive advice," by V. Starck, et al.   NORD MED.   86: 1430-1432, December 2, 1971.

"Seasonality of gonorrhea in the United States," by C. E. Cornelius, III.   HSMHA HEALTH REP.   86:157-160, February, 1971.

"Secondary syphilis with chickenpox in an adult," by

N. J. Fiumara, et al. BR J VENER DIS. 47:142-143, April, 1971.

"Sensitivity and appearance of resistance to rifampicin in N. gonorrhoeae," by I. Juhlin, et al. ACTA PATHOL MICROBIOL. 79:445, 1971.

"Sensitivity and reproducibility of Thayer-Martin culture medium in diagnosing gonorrhea in women," by J. G. Caldwell, et al. AM J OBSTET GYNECOL. 109:463-468, February 1, 1971.

"The sensitivity of gonococci to different antibiotics," by D. Danielsson. LAKARTIDNINGEN. 68:4273-4277 passim, September 15, 1971.

"Sensitivity of Mycoplasma suipneumoniae to penicillin-G," by N. F. Friis. ACTA VET SCAND. 12:120-121, 1971.

"Sensitivity to antibiotics of gonococcal strains isolated from sailors at Rotterdam," by A. Wols-Van der Wielen. BR J VENER DIS. 47:190-191, June, 1971.

"Septic gonococcal dermatitis." BR MED J. 1:472-473, February 27, 1971.

"Septic gonococcal dermatitis," by J. Barr, et al. BR MED J. 1:482-485, February 27, 1971.

"Sequelae of neonatal inclusion conjunctivitis and associated disease in parents," by C. H. Mordhorst, et al. AM J OPHTHALMOL. 71:861-867, April, 1971.

"Sequelae of sexual freedom: the sexually transmitted diseases," by C. S. Nicol. PROC R SOC MED. 64:1108-1111, November, 1971.

"Seriologic and parasitologic survey in aboriginal populations of the Republic of Rwanda. I. Results of the seriologic survey. Frequency of syphilis in aboriginal populations of the Republic of Rwanda. II. Results of the parasitologic survey: protist and filariae," by R. Biemans, et al. BULL SOC PATHOL EXOT. 64:277-291, May-June, 1971.

"Serodiagnosis of candidiasis," by L. Bienias. POL TYG LEK. 26:363-369, March 8, 1971.

"Serologic detection of gonorrhea," by B. B. Diena. ANN INTERN MED. 75:135, July, 1971.

"Serologic diagnosis of lues," by C. Garofoli. POLICLINICO. 78:452-460, June 1, 1971.

"Serologic diagnosis of systemic candidiasis in patients with acute leukemia," by F. Rosener, et al. AM J MED. 51:54-62, July, 1971.

"Serologic syphilis reactions in the Tangiers region," by M. Mailloux. MAROC MED. 51:172-173, March, 1971.

"Serologic tests for syphilis diagnosis in general practice," by I. Rácz. ORV HETIL. 112:630-631, March, 1971.

"Serological study in normal animals," by A. Utrilla. ACTAS DERMOSIFILIOGR. 61:1-12, January-February, 1970.

"Serology of syphilis. Development and concepts. Study on 50 patients," by L. Belli, et al PRENSA MED ARGENT. 58:720-725, June 4, 1971.

"Serology of venereal infections," by J. Meyer-Rohn. Z ALLGEMEINMED. 47:887-890, June 20, 1971.

"Seroresistant syphilis," by N. M. Ovchinnikov. VESTN DERMATOL VENEROL. 45:35-41, August, 1971.

"Serum, lymph node and testicular concentrations of

penicillin in 31 healthy or syphilitic rabbits
treated with penicillin," by J. C. Pechère, et
al. PATHOL BIOL. 19:49-52, January, 1971.

"Sexual activity and cervical carcinoma," by H. J.
Buchsbaum. J IOWA MED SOC. 61:559, September,
1971."

Sexual behaviour of male Pakistanis attending venereal
disease clinics in Great Britain," by A. S. Hossain.
SOC SCI MED. 5:227-241, June, 1971.

"The sexually transmitted diseases," by C. S. Nicol.
PRACTITIONER. 206:277-279, February, 1971.

"Sexually transmitted infections," by V. T. Searle-
Jordan. HUMANIST. 86:262-264, September, 1971.

"Sexually transmitted infections in the schoolchild,"
by J. L. Fluker. MIDWIFE HEALTH VISIT. 6:91-96,
March, 1970.

"She may look clean, but..." EMERGENCY MED. 3:98-
101 plus, March, 1971.

"The significance of cardiolipin immunofluorescence
(CLF)," by J. M. Wright, et al. PROC R SOC MED.
64:419-422, April, 1971.

"Significance of the lymphocyte transformation test in
dermatology," by N. Simon, et al. BERUFSDERNATOSEN.
18:189-219, August, 1970.

"Significance of the Nelson reaction in the diagnosis
of syphilitic organ involvement," by J. Kozakiewicz, et al. POL TYG LEK. 26:706-708, May 10,
1971.

"The silent epidemic--venereal disease," by H. Pariser.
VA MED MON. 98:635-636, December, 1971.

"Silver nitrate and the eyes of the newborn. Crede's

contribution to preventive medicine," by G. B. Forbes, et al. AM J DIS CHILD. 121:1-3, January, 1971.

"A simplified schema for the evaluation of reactive serological tests for syphilis," by L. Nicholas. J CHRONIC DIS. 24:281-284, August, 1971.

"Simultaneous infection of urinary tract and external genital organs in young and adolescent girls," by K. Vesely. GYNECOL PRAT. 22:191-192, 1971.

"Single dose cures 96% of V.D. cases." AM DRUGGIST. 163:62-63, June 14, 1971.

"A 'single dose' treatment of gonococcal urethritis with rifampicin," by V. L. Ongom. BR J VENER DIS. 47:188-189, June, 1971.

"Single-dose treatment of gonorrhoea with penicillin or thiamphenicol and its effect on T. pallidum in experimental syphilis," by D. Petzold. BR J VENER DIS. 47:380, October, 1971.

"Single oral dose ampicillin-probenecid treatment of gonorrhea in the male," by P. A. Kvale, et al. JAMA. 215:1449-1453, March 1, 1971.

"Site of action of efficacy of antisyphilitic treament with penicillin. II. Problems of penicillin dosage," by A. Luger. HAUTARZT. 22:1-6, January, 1971.

"Skin tests in penicillin allergy," by H. Hellenbroich, et al. HAUTARZT. 22:18-24, January, 1971.

"Social antivenereal activity of the Polish Eugenic Society in Warsaw (1916-1939). A contribution to the history of medical societies," by R. Zablotniak. POL MED J. 10:1024-1030, 1971.

"Socio-medical aspects of patients with venereal diseases," by N. Gustavsson. LAKARTIDNINGEN. 68:

4280-4284 passim, September 15, 1971.

"Solid non-agar egg medium for culture of Neisseria," by
M. Pekowski, et al. POL TYG LEK. 26:988-990, June
28, 1971.

"Some enzyme and isoenzyme activities in Trichomonas vaginalis," by M. Chýle, et al. FOLIA MICROBIOL. 16:142-
143, 1971.

"Some enzymes and isoenzymes of Trichomonas vaginalis
and changes in their activities after inoculation
with live mamalian virus," by M. Chýle, et al. CAS
LEK CESK. 110:234-236, March, 1971.

"Some results and prospects of scientific research of
the Department of Dermatologic and Venereal Diseases
of the Tashkent Medical Institute," by A. A. Akovbian.
VESTN DERMATOL VENEROL. 44:3-7, September, 1970.

"Some unusual manifestations of syphilis. Condylomata
lata of the face. A retrospective diagnosis," by V.
N. Sehgal, et al. BR J VENER DIS. 47:204-205, June,
1971.

"Some urgent problems of current syphilidology," by A.
A. Studnitsin, et al. VESTN DERMATOL VENEROL. 45:3-
9, July, 1971.

"Specificity of the FTA-200 test and the FTA-ABS test,"
by B. Evelk. HAUTARZT. 22:442-445, October, 1971.

"Spurious manifestations of cerebral tumor in the course
of hysterical reaction in a child with syphilic encephalopathy," by A. Bratkowa. POL TYG LEK. 26:
217-218, July 8, 1971.

"Squibb's amphotericin B in treatment of Candida albicans and Trichomonas vaginalis infections," by D.
Panaitescu, et al. ARCH ROUM PATHOL EXP MICROBIOL.
30:79-86, March, 1971.

"Stimulation of the catabolism of reserve materials in starved yeast by alcohols and other agents," by W. Rambeck, et al. HOPPE SEYLERS Z PHYSIOL CHEM. 352: 65-70, January, 1971.

"Statement on venereal disease." J KANS MED SOC. 72: 332 passim, July, 1971.

"Sterility in urogenital trichomoniasis," by J. Schmör. WIEN MED WOCHENSCHR. 120:808-812, November 14, 1970.

"Strains of Trichomonas vaginalis resistant to metronidazole," by L. M. Korik. VESTN DERMATOL VENEROL. 45: 77-80, January, 1971.

"Studies on T-strain mycoplasmas in nongonococcal urethritis, " by E. Jansson, et al. BR J VENER DIS. 47: 122-125, April, 1971.

"Studies on Treponema pallidum haemagglutination antibodies. I. TPHA antibodies in experimental syphilitic rabbits," by S. Okamoto, et al. BR J VENER DIS. 47:77-80, April, 1971.

"A study of candida in one thousand and seven women," by F. B. Desmond, et al. NZ MED J. 73:9-13, January, 1971.

"Study of Chlamydiae in patients with lymphogranuloma venereum and urethritis attending a venereal diseases clinic," by R. N. Philip, et al. BR J VENER DIS. 47: 114-121, April, 1971.

"Study of mycoplasma in university students with nongonococcal urethritis," by S. Sueltmann, et al. HEALTH LAB SCI. 8:62-66, April, 1971.

"Study of the trichomonacidal properties of pyrithione (1-hydroxy-2-(1,H)-pyridinethione sodium salt)," by R. Cavier, et al. ANN PHARM FR. 29:211-214, March, 1971.

"Study of 2 cases of congenital syphilitic hepatitis with biopsy," by G. Lepercq, et al. ANN MED INTERNE. 122:633-638, May, 1971.

"Sulphydryl sensitivity of syphilitic antibodies and temperature dependence in complement fixation," by M. Surjan, et al. BR J VENER DIS. 47:87-90, April, 1971.

"Survey of gonorrhoea practices in Great Britain. British Cooperative Clinical Group." BR J VENER DIS. 47: 17-26, February, 1971.

"Susceptibility of the cell walls of some yeasts to lysis by enzymes of Helix pomatia," by J. P. Brown. CAN J MICROBIOL. 17:205-208, February, 1971.

"Symptomatic anorectal gonorrhea in an adolescent female," by W. T. Speck, et al. AM J DIS CHILD. 122: 438-439, November, 1971.

"Syphilis." CALIF MED. 115:47-60, August, 1971.

"Syphilis." CLIN SYMPOSIA. 23,3:3-32, 1971.

"Syphilis," by K. Mizuoka. NAIKA. 27:1256-1260, June, 1971.

"Syphilis among employees of the health service establishments treated at the Department of Dermatology of the Medical Academy in Cracow in 1960-1969." PREZEGL DERMATOL. 58:435-440, 1971.

"Syphilis and gonorrhea at the Munich University dermatological hospital, 1959-1969, " by D. Petzoldt, et al. HAUTARZT. 22:253-257, June, 1971.

"Syphilis and Neanderthal man," by D. J. Wright. NATURE (London). 229:409, February 5, 1971.

"Syphilis diagnosis in the age of antibiotics," by A. Luger. WIEN KLIN WOCHENSCHR. 83:241-245, April

9, 1971.

"Syphilis in the Bible," by L. Goldman. ARCH DERMATOL.
103:535-536, May, 1971.

"Syphilis in the Bundeswehr. Statistical evaluation of
documentations from the past 10 years," by H. Biehler.
HAUTARZT. 22:206-213, May, 1971.

"Syphilis in the Hutten skeleton. Last doubts on the
true identity of the skeleton discovered on the
Ufenau island in Lake Zurich could be dissipated
through research," by H. Jung. HAUTARZT. 22:509,
November, 1971.

"Syphilis lesions of the stomach treated surgically,"
by A. Kulicz, et al. POL PRZEGL CHIR. 43:641-643,
1971.

"Syphilis--1957 to 1970," by J. Murphree. J MED ASSOC
STATE ALA. 40:479-480, January, 1971.

"Syphilis of the aorta in the autopsy material of the
Pathological Institute of the Medical Academy in
Lübeck, in the years 1949-1968," by H. G. Gürich, et
al. ZENTRALBL ALLG PATHOL. 114:499-504, 1971.

"Syphilis reference serology," by A. Fischman, et al.
NZ MED J. 74:238-240, October, 1971.

"Syphilis serodiagnosis, with special reference to FTA-
ABS and TPHA," by H. Ota, et al. J JAP ASSOC IN-
FECT DIS. 45:112-115, March, 1971.

"Syphilitic aortic aneurysm," by J. A. Greenberg. N
ENGL J MED. 284:394, February 18, 1971.

"Syphilitic aortitis in the aged," by P. Armand, et al.
MARS MED. 108:455-458, 1971.

"Syphilitic chorio-retinitis: report of an active case,"
by M. A. Mohamed. BULL OPHTHALMOL SOC EGYPT. 63:

217-221, 1970.

"Syphilitic ostial coronaritis. Analysis of 6 observations," by P. Michaud, et al. J CARDIOVASC SURG. 12:254-263, May-June, 1971.

"Syphilitic pulmonary infarct revealing gumma," by J. Vidal, et al. PRESSE MED. 79:763, April 3, 1971.

"Syphilitic scleritis. Clinical and angiographic aspects," by F. Déodati, et al. BULL SOC OPHTHALMOL FR. 71:63-65, January, 1971.

"T-strains of mycoplasma and nongonococcal urethritis," by H. Haas, et al. BR J VENER DIS. 47:131-134, April, 1971.

"Teaching about venereal diseases in medical schools," by C. J. Alarcón. BOL OF SANIT PANAM. 70:103-111, January, 1971.

"Teaching of dermatologic and venereal diseases at the dental department," by B. M. Pashkov, et al. VESTN DERMATOL VENEROL. 45:68-72, November, 1971.

"Techniques of demonstration of IgM type antibodies in congenital infections," by G. Dropsy, et al. ANN BIOL CLIN. 29:67-73, 1971.

"Temporary positiveness of the F.A.T. test in primary syphilis during the course of treatment," by G. F. Strani, et al. G ITAL DERMATOL. 46:334-335, July, 1971.

"Tertiary syphilis," by R. Degos, et al. BULL SOC FR DERMATOL SYPHILIGR. 78:287-288, 1971.

"Tertiary syphilis of the nasal fossa and the pharynx," by E. Gil Tutor. ACTA OTORINOLARYNGOL IBER AM. 22:366-384, 1971.

"Testing for congenital syphilis in interstitial keratitis," by J. L. Smith. AM J OPHTHALMOL. 72:816-820, October, 1971.

"Testing of blood donors for syphilis," by M. F. Garner, et al. MED J AUST. 1:1374-1376, June 26, 1971.

"Testing of blood donors for syphilis," by M. L. Verso, et al. MED J AUST. 2:281, July 31, 1971.

"Tetracycline in pregnancy?" by B. G. Newman. ANN INTERN MED. 75:648-649, October, 1971.

"Tetracycline inhibition of Mycoplasma ribosomal protein synthesis," by C. C. Fraterrigo, et al. J ANTIBIOT. 24:185-188, March, 1971.

"Therapeutic tips in dermatological practice," by R. Schuppli. DERMATOLOGICA. 142:286-289, 1971.

"Therapy and therapy-control in uncomplicated gonorrhea," by H. Hansson, et al. LAKARTIDNINGEN. 68: 4268-4272, September 15, 1971.

"Therapy for incubating syphilis. Effectiveness of gonorrhea treatment," by A. L. Schroeter, et al. JAMA. 218:711-713, November 1, 1971.

"Therapy for syphilis during pregnancy," by R. P. George, Jr. N ENGL J MED. 284:1271-1272, June 3, 1971.

"Therapy of gonorrhea with tetracycline," by J. Danda, et al. CESK DERMATOL. 46:1-6, February, 1971.

"Therapy of syphilis at the Prague Medical Clinic in the year 1824," by L. Sinkulová. CESK DERMATOL. 46:87-90, April, 1971.

"Therapy of venereal infections," by H. J. Heite. Z ALLGEMEINMED. 47:457-462, March 31, 1971.

"Therapy of viral, mycoplasmal and rickettsial infections,"
by M. W. Rytel, et al. WIS MED J. 70:116-120, April,
1971.

"Thoughts on the treament of vaginitis," by G. W. Gray.
J MED ASSOC STATE ALA. 41:79, August, 1971.

"3 cases of resistance to antisyphilitic treatment," by
KhN Khidyrov, et al. VESTN DERMATOL VENEROL. 44:57-
59, September, 1970.

"Thrush colpitis," by G. K. Döring. DTSCH MED WOCHEN-
SCHR. 96:358, February 19, 1971.

"Thymic conversion of Candida albicans from commensalism
to pathogenism," by E. P. Schoch, Jr. ARCH DERMATOL.
103:311-319, March, 1971.

"To fight V.D." J PRACT NURS. 21:13, March, 1971.

"Today's values; how can we stop the spread of venereal
disease?" by E. McConnell. FORECAST HOME ECON. 17:
F30-31, November, 1971.

"Transfer of gonococcal urethritis from man to chimpanzee. An animal model for gonorrhea," by C. T.
Lucas, et al. JAMA. 216:1612-1614, June 7, 1971.

"Transgrow, a medium for transport and growth of Neisser-
ia gonorrhoeae and Neisseria meningitidis," by J. E.
Martin, Jr., et al. HSMHA HEALTH REP. 86:30-33,
January, 1971.

"Transmission possibilities of gonorrhea?" by H. Götz.
MUNCH MED WOCHENSCHR. 113:742-743, May 7, 1971.

"Transport of herpes simplex virus in Stuart's medium,"
by P. Rodin, et al. BR J VENER DIS. 47:198-199,
June, 1971.

"Transverse septum formation in budding cells of the
yeastlike fungus Candida albicans," by J. L. Shan-

non, et al. J BACTERIOL. 106:1026-1028, June, 1971.

"Treatment and prevention of syphilis and gonorrhea."
MED LETT DRUGS THER. 13:85-87, October, 1971.

"Treatment of Bartholin cysts," by G. Vlasis. AM FAM
PHYSICIAN. 3:85-86, June, 1971.

"Treatment of candidal vulvovaginitis and urethritis
with 1 per cent alcohol-water solution of levorin,"
by I. I. Shkliar, et al. VESTN DERMATOL VENEROL.
45:81-84, February, 1971.

"Treatment of early syphilis and venereal lymphogranu-
lomatosis with doxycyclines," by H. Hevia, et al.
REV MED CHIL. 99:402-405, June, 1971.

"Treatment of gonorrhea," by L. J. Lancaster. JAMA.
217:1106, August 23, 1971.

"Treatment of gonorrhea," by F. L. Roberts. JAMA. 218:
446, October 18, 1971.

"Treatment of gonorrhea in women with Doxycycline," by
J. Bartunek. MED WELT. 14:504-505, April 3, 1971.

"Treatment of gonorrhea in young girls," by M. Loza-
Tulimowska, et al. PRZEGL DERMATOL. 58:183-186,
March-April, 1971.

"Treatment of gonorrhoea with aqueous benzyl penicillin
plus probenecid," by A. M. Niordson, et al. ACTA
DERM VENEROL. 51:311-314, 1971.

"Treatment of gonorrhoea with single oral doses. Results obtained with doxycycline or rifampicin compared with intramuscular penicillin," by E. P. van
Steenbergen. BR J VENER DIS. 47:111-113, April, 1971.

"Treatment of gonorrhea with sulphamethoxazole-trimethoprim," by H. Svindland. TIDSSKR NOR LAEGEFOREN. 91:
1753-1755, August 30, 1971.

"Treatment of gonorrhoea with two oral doses of antibiotics. Trials of cephalexin and of triple tetracycline, (Deteclo)," by R. R. Wilcoz. BR J VENER DIS. 47:31-33, February, 1971.

"Treatment of gynecologic infection by combined tetracycline and amphotericin B," by M. Van Gijsegem. BRUX MED. 51:391-393, May, 1971.

"Treatment of neurosyphilis," by J. Tempski-Templehof, et al. HAREFUAH. 80:196-198, February 15, 1971.

"Treatment of prostatitis," by D. Volter. DTSCH MED WOCHENSCHR. 96:1091-1093, June 18, 1971.

"Treatment of trichomonas infections with tinidazol in women," by J. Diwald. WIEN MED WOCHENSCHR. 121: 492-494, June 12, 1971.

"Treatment of trichomoniasis vaginalis," by H. Heiss. WIEN MED WOCHENSCHR. 121:30-33, January 16, 1971.

"Treatment of trichomoniasis in the female with a 5-day course of metronidazole (Flagyl)," by A. N. McClean. BR J VENER DIS. 47:36-37, February, 1971.

"Treatment of uncomplicated gonorrhea with a one time dose of doxycycline," by H. Hammar, et al. LAKAR-TIDNINGEN. 68:4278-4279, September 15, 1971.

"Treatment of uncomplicated gonorrhea with a single oral dose of doxycycline," by S. Liden, et al. ACTA DERM VENEROL. 51:221-224, 1971.

"Treatment of vaginal fluor," by G. Kümmel. MED WELT. 2:65-66, January 9, 1971.

"Treatment of vaginal inflammation with metronidazole," by K. Suk, et al. ZENTRALBL GYNAEKOL. 93:1380-1383, October 2, 1971.

"Treatment of vaginal trichomoniasis with takimetol tablets (metronidazole preparation) SANFUJINKA JISSAI. 20:99-103, January, 1971.

"Treatment of vaginitis of diverse etiology with pimaricin," by F. Bianchi. MINERVA GINECOL. 23:489-492, May 31, 1971.

"Treatment of venereal diseases," by M. Janner. Z ALLGEMEINMED. 47:891-899, June 20, 1971.

"Treatment possibilities in fluor genitalis in dermatological practice," by H. Weitgasser. Z HAUT GESCHLECHTSKR. 46:107-110, February 15, 1971.

"Trends and status of gonorrhea in the United States," by W. J. Brown J INFECT DIS. 123:682-688, June, 1971.

"Treponema pallidum immobilization test in properly treated patients with syphilis," by T. V. Vasil'ev, et al. VESTN DERMATOL VENEROL. 45:52-57, June, 1971.

"Trial of Situdicine in gynecologic therapy," by M. Bruhat, et al. LYON MED. 225:773-775, April 25, 1971.

"A trial in treatment of gonorrhea with a sulphonamide with prolonged effect (sulfapherin)," by B. L. Jorgensen. UGESKR LAEGER. 133:1257-1258, July 2, 1971.

"Trichomonas and oxytetracycline," by S. Szanto. BR MED J. 2:467, May 22, 1971.

"Trichomoniasis in a closed community: Efficacy of metronidazole," by E. E. Keighley. BR MED J. 1:207-209, January 23, 1971.

"Trichomoniasis of the paranasal sinuses," by E. Teisanu, et al. OTORINOLARINGOLOGIE. 16:265-269, July-August, 1971.

"Trimethoprim for the prevention of overgrowth by swarming Proteus in the cultivation of gonococci,"

by K. Odegaard. ACTA PATHOL MICROBIOL SCAND. 79:
545-548, 1971.

"Trimeththoprim-sulphamethoxazole in gonorrhoea," by
S. Ullman, et al. ACTA DERM VENEREOL. 51:394-
396, 1971.

"Trimethoprim-sulphammethoxazole (Septrin) in the treatment of rectal gonorrhoea," by M. A. Waugh. BR J
VENER DIS. 47:34-35, February, 1971.

"2 cases of vaginitis due to an as yet unknown parasite
in gynecologic pathology," by M. Gaudefroy, et al.
J SCI MED LILLE. 89:301-302, August-September, 1971

"2 rare cases of secondary syphilis," by M. F. Roitburd.
VESTN DERMATOL VENEROL. 44:76-79, November, 1970.

"Ulcus molle in a woman," by H. R. Manuel, et al. NED
TIJDSCHR GENEESKD. 115:71, January 9, 1971.

"Ultrastructure of Treponema pallidum Nichols following
lysis by physical and chemical methods. I. Enve-
lope, wall, membrane and fibrils," by S. Jackson, et
al. ARCH MIKROBIOL. 76:308-324, 1971.

  --II. Axial filaments," by S. Jackson, et al. ARCH
MIKROBIOL. 76:325-340, 1971.

"Uncomplicated gonorrhea treated with Trimethoprim
and sulphamethoxazol," by B. L. Jorgensen, et al.
UGESKR LAEGER. 133:1259-1260, July 2, 1971

"The unmentionable diseases," by K. Dicker. NURS
TIMES. 67:94 plus, January 21, 1971.

"Unsuccessful treatment of early symptomatic syphilis
following oral administration of detreomycin, erythromycin and oxyterracin," by J. Lebioda, et al. PRZEGL
LEK. 27:469-472, 1971.

"An unusual Jarisch-Herxheimer reaction," by R. N. Thin.
BR J VENER DIS. 47:293-294, August, 1971.

"Urethritis in male children," by D. I. Williams, et al.
PROC R SOC MED. 64:133-134, February, 1971.

"Use of single doses of thiamphenicol in gonococcal urethritis," by V. Rodrigues, et al. REV BRAS MED.
28:288-290, June, 1971.

"Use of transport media in the cultural diagnosis of
gonorrhea," by M. V. Iatsukha. VESTN DERMATOL
VENEROL. 45:58-61, November, 1971.

"The usefulness of immediate skin tests to haptenes
derived from penicillin. A study in patients with
a history of previous adverse reactions to penicillin," by M. J. Fellner, et al. ARCH DERMATOL. 103:
371-374, April, 1971.

"Using one dose of doxycycline or penicillin to treat
men with gonococcal urethritis," by S. R. Jones,
et al. HSMHA HEALTH REP. 86:849-854, September,
1971.

"V.D." by A. Blanzaco. TODAYS EDUC. 60:41, December,
1971.

"V.D." by H. Miller. LISTENER. 86:572, October 28,
1971.

"V.D.: the clock is ticking," by M. Strage. TODAY"S
HEALTH. 49:16-18 plus, April, 1971.

"V.D.: Gonorrhea incidence put at 2 million annually

in U. S." HOSP PRACT. 6:27 plus, June, 1971.

V.D.: a national epidemic." MED TIMES. 99:109 passim, May, 1971.

"V.D. statistics," by A. S. Wigfield. BR MED J. 4: 750, December 18, 1971.

"The VDRL slide test in 322 cases of darkfield positive primary syphilis," by R. D. Wende, et al. SOUTH MED J. 64:633-634, May, 1971.

"Vaginal aspirate studies in children. An atraumatic method," by V. J. Capraro, et al. OBSTET GYNECOL. 37:462-464, March, 1971.

"Vaginal candidiasis treated with nystatin containing globules," by T. Lakos. ORV HETIL. 112:1712-1714, July 18, 1971.

"Vaginal infections and infestations diagnosed by cytology," by E. Gutiérrez Valverde, et al. GINECOL OBSTET MEX. 30:619-625, December, 1971.

"Vaginal moniliasis during pregnancy and during intake of oral contraceptives," by W. Gruber, et al. WIEN MED WOCHENSCHR. 120:898-900, November 28, 1970.

"Vaginal yeast growth and contraceptive practices," by W. N. Spellacy, et al. OBSTET GYNECOL. 38:343-349, September, 1971.

"Vaginitis and tights," by J. Stallworthy. BR MED J. 2:108, April 10, 1971.

"Validity of the VDRL test on cerebrospinal fluid contaminated by blood," by N. N. Izzat, et al. BR J VENER DIS. 47:162-164, June, 1971.

"The value of autoantibodies to vascular lipids in syphilis and non-syphilis," by O. J. Stone. INT J DERMATOL. 10:31-34, January-March, 1971.

"Value of present-day serological tests in the diagnosis
of symptomless sources of infection and contacts in
early syphilis," by W. Manikowska-Lesińska, et al.
PRZEGL DERMATOL. 58:157-162, March-April, 1971.

"Value of the Treponema pallidum immobilization test in
the detection of late and visceral syphilis in general hospital patients," by N. M. Ovchinnikov, et al.
VESTN DERMATOL VENEROL. 45:53-57, September, 1971.

"Value of vaginal and rectal cultures in the diagnosis
of gonorrhoea. With special reference to areas with
limited medical facilities," by G. A. Olsen. BR J
VENER DIS. 47:102-106, April, 1971.

"Venereal disease." SOUTH MED J. 64:1157-1158, September, 1971.

"Venereal disease," by F. W. Barton. JAMA. 216:1472-
1473, May 31, 1971.

"Venereal disease," by T. H. Bierre. OCCUP HEALTH.
4:3-4, December, 1970.

"Venereal disease," by D. Rubin. McCALLS. 98:64
plus, June, 1971.

"Venereal disease. Acquired syphilis--drugs and blood
test," by W. J. Brn. AM J NURS. 71:713-715, April,
1971.

"Venereal disease. Communities strike back," by W. F.
Schwartz. AM J NURS. 71:724, April, 1971.

"Venereal disease. TLC with the penicillin," by R.
Matthews. AM J NURS. 71:720-723, April, 1971..

"Venereal disease. Women, the unwitting carriers of
gonorrhea," by P. E. Lenz. AM J NURS. 71:716-
719, April, 1971.

"The venereal disease dilemma: A case in question,"

by S. J. Bender. J SCH HEALTH. 41:105-107, February, 1971.

"Venereal disease education," by M. Riggs. CALIF MED. 115:74-75, October, 1971.

"Venereal disease education program." ROCKY MT MED J. 68:28, December, 1971.

"Venereal disease education using a teaching question-naire, by R. M. Manuel, et al. CAN J PUBLIC HEALTH. 62:336-339, July-August, 1971.

"Venereal disease: the enemy is us," edited by M. F. Doherty, et al. NY STATE ED. 58:19-27, March, 1971.

"Venereal disease in teen-agers," by H. M. Wallace. CLIN OBSTET GYNECOL. 14:432-441, June, 1971.

"Venereal disease in women. I." by C. S. Nichol. BR MED J. 2:328-329, May 8, 1971.

--II." by C. S. Nicol. BR MED J. 2:383-384, May 15, 1971.

"Venereal disease of the anal region," by R. K. Menda, et al. DIS COLON RECTUM. 14:454-459, November-December, 1971.

"Venereal disease pandemic," by C. Roberts, et al. N.Y. TIMES MAG. November 7, 1971, p. 62 plus.

"Venereal disease problem in Canada," by S. E. Acres, et al CAN NURSE. 67:24-27, July, 1971.

"Venereal disease rampant." JAMA. 218:731, November 1, 1971.

"Venereal disease research; slow progress." CHEM & ENG N. 49:46-48 plus, June 21, 1971.

"Venereal granuloma," by O. Mattos, et al. REV BRAS

MED. 28:265, June, 1971.

"Venereal diseases." BORD MED. 4:479-480, February, 1971.

"Venereal diseases." LANCET. 1:691-692, April 3, 1971.

"Venereal diseases. A study of the attitudes toward and knowledge of them among young people," by J. Wallin. LAKARTIDNINGEN. 68:199-205, January, 1971.

"Venereal diseases and modern contraception," by M. Vojta. CESK GYNEKOL. 36:60-61, February, 1971.

"Venereal diseases as a problem of national and international health. Problem of control of gonorrhea," by Á. Campos Salas. SALUD PUBLICA MEX. 13:41-52, January-February, 1971.

"Venereal diseases at present," by W. Burckhardt. PRAXIS 60:408-411, March 30, 1971.

"Venereal diseases in Lagos," by T. Daramola, et al. ISR J MED SCI. 7:288-294, February, 1971.

"Venereal diseases-new problems for the physician and the community," by A. J. Dalzell-Ward. DISEASE-A-MONTH. January, 1971, p. 1-45.

"Venereal infection." MIDWIFE HEALTH VISIT. 7:173, May, 1971.

"Venerologic importance of mycoplasmas," by A. Horváth, et al. ORV HETIL. 112:1820-1822, August 1, 1971.

"A venereological view of the prostate gland," by L. Molin. LAKARTIDNINGEN. 68:3500-3504, July 28, 1971.

"Viral carcinogenesis in venereally susceptible organs," by A. Ravich. CANCER. 27:1493-1496, June, 1971.

"Virulence factors in gonococci." DTSCH MED WOCHENSCHR. 96:137, January 15, 1971.

"Witkop disease. Two 'favoid' cases due to syphilis," by P. S. Jain. BR J VENER DIS. 47:216-217, June, 1971.

"World-wide epidemiological tendencies of syphilis and blenorrhagia," by T. Guthe. BOL OF SANIT PANAM. 70: 6-25, January, 1971.

"The X in sex." NURS TIMES. 67:380-381, April 1, 1971.

"Yaws," by I. Kantor, et al. ARCH DERMATOL. 103:546-547, May, 1971.

"Yaws, mycoplasma pneumoniae and cold agglutinins in New Guineans," by P. B. Booth. MED J AUST. 1:715, March 27, 1971.

"Yaws, mycoplasma pneumoniae and cold agglutinins in New Guineans," by J. Kariks. MED J AUST. 1:85-87, January 9, 1971.

"Yeast fungus infection of the urinary tract," by J. Schönebeck, et al NORD MED. 85:188, February 11, 1971.

PERIODICAL LITERATURE

SUBJECT INDEX

AMERICAN MEDICAL ASSOCIATION
"AMA statement on venereal disease." MO MED. 68:604,
August, 1971.

"Doctor's attention urged by AMA council to problems
of VD." MICH MED. 70:648, July, 1971.

AMPHOTERICIN B
"Squibb's amphotericin B in treatment of Candida albicans and Trichomonas vaginalis infections," by D.
Panaitescu, et al. ARCH ROUM PATHOL EXP MICROBIOL.
30:79-86, March, 1971.

"Treatment of gynecologic infection by combined tetracycline and amphotericin B," by M. Van Gijsegem.
BRUX MED. 51:391-393, May, 1971.

AMPICILLIN
"Ampicillin in the treatment of gonorrheal salpingitis,"
by E. Hedberg, et al. LAKARTIDNINGEN. 68:335-340,
January 20, 1971.

"Clinical trials with ampicillin in the treatment of
gonorrheal urethritis in males," by S. Arap. HOSPI-
TAL 77:1173-1177, April, 1970.

"In vitro studies on the mechanism of penicillin and
ampicillin drug reactions," by Z. H. Haddad, et al.

INT ARCH ALLERGY APPL IMMUNOL (Basel). 41:72-78, 1971

"One-day oral ampicillin-treatment of gonorrhea in young adults," by L. H. Shapiro, et al. OBSTET GYNECOL. 37:414-418, March, 1971.

"Oral ampicillin in uncomplicated gonorrhea. 3. Result of treatment in women with positive rectal culture," by G. Eriksson. ACTA DERM VENEREOL. 51:305-310, 1971.

"Oral ampicillin in uncomplicated gonorrhea. 4. Comparison of pharmacological and clinical results," by G. Eriksson. ACTA DERM VENEREOL. 51:467-475, 1971.

"Oral single-dose treatment of male and female gonorrhea with ampicillin alone and combined with probenecid," by A. Bro-Jorgensen, et al   UGESKR LAEGER. 133: 1253-1256, July 2, 1971.

"Reduced maternal plasma and urinary estriol during ampicillin treatment," by K. Willman, et al. AM J OBSTET GYNECOL. 109:893-896, March 15, 1971.

"Single dose cures 96% of VD cases." AM DRUGGIST. 163: 62-63, June 14, 1971.

"Single oral dose ampicillin-probenecid treatment of gonorrhea in the male," by P. A. Kvale, et al   JAMA. 215:1449-1453, March 1, 1971.

ANO-RECTAL VENEREAL DISEASES
"Anal venereal diseases in two practices. (1958-1968)," by J. Rivoire, et al. AM J PROCTOL. 22:189-190, June, 1971.

"The dermatologist and pruritus ani," by J. E. Racouchot

ANO-RECTAL VENEREAL DISEASES

et al. AM J PROCTOL. 22:191-195, June, 1971.

"Venereal disease of the anal region," by R. K. Menda,
et al. DIS COLON RECTUM. 14:454-459, November -
December, 1971.

ARTHRITIS
"Arthritis, vaginitis and cardiac murmur," by S. Jacobs.
J LA STATE MED SOC 123:179-182, May, 1971.

"A case of combined inflammatory rheumatic and neuro-
pathic joint changes," by O. Erhart, et al. Z
ORTHOP. 107:676-682, May, 1970.

BALANITIS AND BALANOPOSTHITIS
"Case of balanoposthitis trichomonadosa," by Z.
Gwiezdzinski, et al. POL TYG LEK. 26:642-643, April
26, 1971.

"Clinical evaluation of carbenoxolone in balanitis,"
by G. W. Csonka, et al. BR J VENER DIS (London).
47:179-181, June, 1971.

"A combination of primary syphilis and trichomononal
balanoposthitis," by E. L. Fridman. VESTN DERMATOL
VENEROL. 45:67-69, 1971.

BAY B 5097
"Bay B 5097, a new orally applicable antifungal sub-
stance with broadspectrum activity. Preliminary and
laboratory experiences in children," by W. Marget,
et al. ACTA PAEDIATR SCAND. 60:341-345, May, 1971.

BEDSONIAE
"Complement-fixing antibodies to Bedsonia in Reiter's
syndrome, TRIC agent infection, and control groups,"
by J Schachter. AM J OPHTHALMOL. 71:857-860,
April, 1971.

BEETHOVEN'S DISEASE

"Beethoven's disease," by K. Herrero Duclaux. PRENSA M
ARGENT. 57:2018-2025, January 1, 1971.

BEJEL
"Bejel or non-venereal endemic syphilis," by M. W.
Kanan, et al. BR J DERMATOL. 84:461-464, May, 1971.

BICILLIN
"Bicillin-6 therapy of gonorrhea in men," by V. E.
Grigoriev, et al. VESTN DERMATOL VENEROL. 45:74-
77, January, 1971.

"Continuous treatment of early forms of syphilis with
penicillin and bicillin," by IuF Korolev. VOEN MED
ZH. 7:76-77, 1971.

"Effect of penicillin and bicillin-1 in experimental
syphilis in rabbits," by N. M. Ovchinnikov, et al.
VESTN DERMATOL VENEROL. 45:42-47, June, 1971.

"Immediate results of bicillin-5 treatment of patients
with infectious forms of syphilis," by S. H. Khamido
VESTN DERMATOL VENEROL. 45:41-44, August, 1971.

"Late results of treating syphilis with bicillin-1,3,4,
and bicillin-3,4 in combination with pyrogenal,"
by T. V. Vasil'ev. VESTN DERMATOL VENEROL. 45:50-
58, January, 1971.

BIOTIN
"Effect of biotin on growth of Candida tropicalis K-41
and synthesis of vitamin B complex," by E. I. Kvasnikov, et al. MIKROBIOL ZH. 33:240-243, March -
April, 1971.

BLENNORRHAGIA
"Bactrim (trimethoprim-sulfamethoxazole) treatment of
female blennorrhagia," by C. B. Schofield, et al.
REV COLOMB OBSTET GINECOL. 22:269-273, July - Augus

BLENNORRHAGIA

1971.

"Current aspects of blennorrhagia. Statistical study
of 200 patients," by P. Amblard, et al. BULL SOC
FR DERMATOL SYPHILIGR. 78:188-190, 1971.

"Keratodermia blennorrhagica in Reiter's disease," by
R. Howell. BR MED J. 1:725-726, March 27, 1971.

"Problems in the control of blennorrhagia," by S. A.
Campos. BOL OF SANIT PANAM. 70:66-78, January,
1971.

"World-wide epidemiological tendencies of syphilis
and blennorhagia," by T. Guthe. BOL OF SANIT
PANAM. 70:6-25, January, 1971.

BLOOD DONORS AND TRANSFUSIONS
"Brucellosis and syphilis transmitted by transfusion,"
by A. Becerra-Garcia. GAC MED MEX. 101:699-701,
June, 1971.

"Possibility of the transmission of syphilis in the
blood of a donor with a latent form of this disease,"
by A. A. Mikhailova, et al. PROBL GEMATOL PERELIV
KROVI. 16:50-51, July, 1971.

"Testing of blood donors for syphilis," by M. F. Garner,
et al. MED J AUST. 1:1374-1376, June 26, 1971.

"Testing of blood donors for syphilis," by M. L. Verso,
et al. MED J AUST. 2:281, July 31, 1971.

CANCER AND PRE-CANCER
"Genital herpes and cervical cancer," by P. Leinikki,
et al. DUODECIM. 87:181-183, 1971.

"Genital herpes and cervical cancer," by A. Singer.
BR MED J. 1:458, February 20, 1971.

CANCER AND PRE-CANCER

"Herpesvirus antibody and carcinoma in situ of the cervix," by L. W. Catalano, et al. JAMA. 217: 447-450, July 26, 1971.

"Relationship of herpes simplex genital infection and carcinoma of the cervix: population studies," by Y. M. Centifanto, et al. AM J OBSTET GYNECOL. 110: 690-692, July 1, 1971.

"Sexual activity and cervical carcinoma," by H. J. Buchsbaum. J IOWA MED SOC. 61:559, September, 1971.

"Viral carcinogenesis in venereally susceptible organs," by A. Ravich. CANCER. 27:1493-1496, June, 1971.

CANDIDA AND CANDIDIASIS

"Acute disseminated and chronic mucocutaneous candidiasis," by P. G. Quie, et al. SEMIN HERMATOL. 8:227-242, July, 1971.

"Alkane oxidation by a particulate preparation from Candida," by C. M. Liu, et al. J BACTERIOL. 106: 830-834, June, 1971.

"Alternate methods of nutrient dosing in continuous phased culture," by P. S. Dawson, et al. CAN J MICROBIOL. 17:435-439, April, 1971.

"Antimicrobial activity of sodium n-alkylsalicylates," by D. Buckley, et al. APPL MICROBIOL. 21:565-568, April, 1971.

"An assessment of the role of Candida albicans and food yeasts in chronic urticaria," by J. James, et al. BR J DERMATOL. 84:227-237, March, 1971.

"Candida and candidiasis," by P. J. Kozinn, et al. JAMA. 217:965-966, August 16, 1971.

"Candida at Boston City Hospital. Clinical and epidemiological characteristics and susceptibility to eight antimicrobial agents," by P. Toala, et al. ARCH INTERN MED. 126:983-989, December, 1970.

"Candidiasis: colonization vs. infection." JAMA. 215: 285-286, January 11, 1971.

"Changes in phosphorus composition of Canida utilis during the cell cycle and postcycle period," by H. Glättli, et al. CAN J MICROBIOL. 17:339-345, March, 1971.

"Demonstration of the antifungal effect of Candistatin paste, a new nystatin preparation, after storage," by J. O. Toyosi, et al. MYKOSEN. 14:145-147, March 1, 1971.

"Demonstration of the inhibitory effect of blood on respiration of Candida albicans using Warburg's apparatus," by J. Kapell, et al. ARCH HYG BAKTERIOL 154:524-532, April, 1971.

"Diagnostic criteria in candidiasis," by L. Bienias. POL TYG LEK. 26:222-225, July 8, 1971.

"Diaper thrush," by W. Gschwandtner, et al. Z HAUT GESCHLECHTSKR. 46:179-183, March 15, 1971.

"Effect of biotin on growth of Candida tropicalis K-41 and synthesis of vitamin B complex," by E. I. Kvasnikov, et al. MIKROBIOL ZH. 33:240-243, March - April, 1971.

"Effect of nystatin on mycelial transformation of Candida albicans cells in the human serum," by H. Buluk, et al. MED DOSW MIKROBIOL. 23:175-181, 1971.

"Effect of pyrimidine derivatives on the formation of

anti-Candida immunity," by E. N. Bol'shakova. ZH
MIKROBIOL EPIDEMIOL IMMUNOBIOL. 48:59-61, February,
1971.

"Enzymatic oxidation of hydrocarbons in Candida inter-
media cells," by L. A. Levchenko, et al. BIOKHIMJIA.
36:88-91, January - February, 1971.

"Epidemiologic associations between vaginal candidiasis
in the pregnant woman and oral thrush in newborn
infants," by A. M. Dolgopol'skala, et al. VOPR OKHR
MATERIN DET. 16:50-54, February, 1971.

"Estimation of dermatophytes (ringworm fungi) and
candida spores in the environment," by Y. M. Clayton,
et al. J MED MICROBIOL. 4:3-4, May, 1971.

"Experimental ascending Candida infections in the
urinary tract," by M. Hatala, et al. CAS LEK CESK.
110:553-558, June 11, 1971.

"Experimental cutaneous Candida albicans infection in
guinea-pigs," by J. Van Cutsem, et al. SABOURAUDIA.
9:17-20, March, 1971.

"An experimental investigation of farmer's lung. Comparative study of the pulmonary clearance capacity
for Aspergillus fumigatus, Candida albicans and
Mycropolyspora faeni in guinea pigs," by C. Voisin,
et al. REV FR ALLERGOL. 11:129-136, April - June,
1971.

"Experimental pathology of pathogenic fungi. Microscopic detectable pathological changes in Candida
albicans due to pimaricin," by H. Rieth. MYKOSEN.
14:47-48, January 1, 1971.

"Fatty acid and hydrocarbon hydroxylation in yeast:
role of cytochrome P-450 in Candida tropicalis," by

J. M. Lebeault, et al. BIOCHEM BIOPHYS RES COMMUN. 42:413-419, February 5, 1971.

"5-fluorocytosine and urinary candidiasis," by R. R. Davies, et al. BR MED J. 1:577-579, March 13, 1971.

"5-fluorocytosine in the treatment of cryptococcal and candida mycoses," by R. J. Fass, et al. ANN INTERN MED. 74:535-539, April, 1971.

"Focal fungal infections treated by immunological therapy with emphasis on vaginal moniliasis," by H. Hosen. TEX MED. 67:56-58, October, 1971.

"Further studies of the germ-tube test for Candida albicans identification," by C. T. Dolan, et al. AM J CLIN PATHOL. 55:733-734, June, 1971.

"A glutinous rice culture medium for demonstration of chlamydospores of Candida albicans," by S. Sukroongreung. MYCOPATHOL MYCOL APPL. 43:329-335, March 25, 1971.

"Growth models of cultures with two liquid phases. V. Substrate dissolved in dispersed phase--experimental observations," by A. Prokop, et al. BIOTECHNOL BIOENG. 13:241-256, March, 1971.

"Identification of Candida isolated from the cutaneous candidiasis by the combined use of confirmatory medium and slide agglutination with monofactorial antibodies," by T. Nishikawa, et al. MYCOPATHOL MYCOL APPL. 43:269-277, March 25, 1971.

"Immunofluorescence studies of candida in human reticuloendothelial phagocytes: implications for immunogenesis and pathogenesis of systemic candidiasis," by C. L. Taschdjian, et al. AM J CLIN PATHOL. 56:50-58, July 8, 1971.

"In vitro studies with the antimycoticum chlortritylimidazole," by W. Ritzerfeld, et al. INT Z KLIN TOXIKOL. 4:204-206, February, 1971.

"The indirect immunofluorescence in the serologic diagnosis of systemic candidiasis," by R. Negroni, et al. MYCOPATHOL MYCOL APPL. 43:355-359, March 25, 1971.

"Indirect immunofluorescence reaction in the serodiagnosis of candidiasis," by L. Bienias. MYKOSEN. 14:115-118, March 1, 1971.

"Influence of gestogenic contraceptive pills on vaginal candidosis," by R. D. Catterall. BR J VENER DIS. 47:45-47, February, 1971.

"Influence of oral contraception upon the occurence of Candida albicans in the vagina," by H. Thulin. NORD MED. 85:399-401, April, 1971.

"Intertriginous and genital Candida mycoses," by W. Meinhof. DTSCH MED WOCHENSCHR. 96:887, May 14, 1971

"Mating responses in Candida lipolytica," by A. I. Herman. J BACTERIOL. 107:371, July, 1971.

"Mechanism of uptake of liquid hydrocarbons by microorganisms," by F. Yoshida, et al. BIOTECHNOL BIOENG. 13:215-228, March, 1971.

"A medium for the diagnosis of vaginal candidiasis," by H. Becker, et al. MYKOSEN. 14:127-130, March 1, 1971.

"Methionine biosynthesis in Candida albicans. I. S-adenosyl-L-methionine (or S-methyl-L-methionine): homocysteine methyltransferase in cell-free extracts from yeast like cells," by D. N. Mardon, et al. CAN

J MICROBIOL. 17:795-802, June, 1971.

"Modification of the composition and structure of the
yeast cell wall by culture in the presence of sulfur
amino acids," by K. A. Killick. J BACTERIOL. 106:
931-937, June, 1971.

"Morphologic and histochemical changes in the mucosa
of the urogenital tract in gonorrhea, trichomonas
and candidiasis," by V. G. Bilik, et al. VESTN
DERMATOL VENEROL. 45:50-53, May, 1971.

"New data on the spore tubule formation of Candida
albicans in various human and animal serums," by
J. O. Toyosi, et al. MYKOSEN. 14:49-51, January
1, 1971.

"Occurence of two maximum temperatures for growth in
yeasts," by A. Oliveira-Baptista, et al. Z ALLG
MIKROBIOL. 11:59-61, 1971.

"Oxytetracycline-nystatin in the prevention of candidal
vaginitis," by M. Silverman, et al. AM J OBSTET
GYNECOL. 111:398-404, October 1, 1971.

"Prevention of vaginal Candida proliferation by the
use of Pimafucin vaginal tablets during metronidazole
treatment," by I. Alteras. BRUX MED. 51:501-503,
July, 1971.

"Rapid identification of yeasts of the Candida albicans
and Candida tropicalis specific by slide agglutination
with species serum," by M. Sefer, et al. ROM MED
REV. 15:8-10, January - March, 1971.

"The reaction of the isoenzymes of transaldolase with
chlorodinitrobenzene," by O. Tsolas, et al. ARCH
BIOCHEM BIOPHYS. 143:516-525, April, 1971.

"Relationship of Torulopsis to candida," by B. G. Leask, et al. LANCET. 1:1300-1301, June 19, 1971.

"Scanning electron microscopic studies of Candida albicans," by W. G. Barnes, et al. J BACTERIOL. 106:276-280, April, 1971

"Serodiagnosis of candidiasis," by L. Bienias. POL TYG LEK. 26:363-369, March 8, 1971.

"Serologic diagnosis of systemic candidiasis in patients with acute leukemia," by F. Rosener, et al. AM J MED. 51:54-62, July, 1971.

"Squibb's amphotericin B in treatment of Candida albicans and Trichomonas vaginalis infections," by D. Panaitescu, et al. ARCH ROUM PATHOL EXP MICRO-BIOL. 30:79-86, March, 1971.

"Stimulation of the catabolism of reserve materials in starved yeast by alcohols and other agents," by W. Rambeck, et al. HOPPE SEYLERS Z PHYSIOL CHEM. 352: 65-70, January, 1971

"A study of candida in one thousand and seven women," by F. B. Desmond, et al. NZ MED J. 73:9-13, January, 1971.

"Susceptibility of the cell walls of some yeasts to lysis by enzymes of Helix pomatia," by J. P. Brown. CAN J MICROBIOL. 17:205-208, February, 1971.

"Thymic conversion of Candida albicans from commensalism to pathogenism," by E. P. Schoch, Jr. ARCH DERMATOL. 103:311-319, March, 1971

"Transverse septum formation in budding cells of the yeastlike fungus Candida albicans," by J. L. Shannon et al. J BACTERIOL. 106:1026-1028, June, 1971.

CANDIDA AND CANDIDIASIS

"Treatment of candidal vulvovaginitis and urethritis with 1 per cent alcohol-water solution of levorin," by I. I. Shkliar, et al. VESTN DERMATOL VENEROL. 45:81-84, February, 1971

"Vaginal candidiasis treated with nystatin containing globules," by T. Lakos. ORV HETIL. 112:1712-1714, July 18, 1971.

"Vaginal moniliasis during pregnancy and during intake of oral contraceptives," by W. Gruber, et al. WIEN MED WOCHENSCHR. 120:898-900, November 28, 1970.

CANDICIDIN
"Pyrolysis-gas chromatography of polyene antifungal antibiotics: the nature of candicidin, levorin, and trichomycin," by H. J. Burrows, et al. J CHROMATOGR. 53:566-571, December 23, 1971.

CANDIDINE
"Exploration of delayed cutaneous hypersensitivity to candidine in newborn and young infants," by R. Carron, et al. PEDIATRIE. 26:259-264, April - May, 1971.

CANDISTATIN
"Demonstration of the antifungal effect of Candistatin paste, a new nystatin preparation, after storage," by J. O. Toyosi, et al. MYKOSEN. 14:145-147, March 1, 1971.

CARBENOXOLONE
"Clinical evaluation of carbenoxolone in balanitis," by G. W. Csonka, et al. BR J VENER DIS. 47:179-181, June, 1971.

CEPHALEXIN
"Treatment of gonorrhea with two oral doses of anti-biotics. Trials of cephalexin and of triple tetra-

CEPHALEXIN

cycline (Deteclo)," by R. R. Willcox. BR J VENER
DIS. 47:31-33, February, 1971.

CEPHALOSPORINS
"Cephalosporin antibiotics in venereal disease," by W.
C. Duncan, et al. POSTGRAD MED J. 47:119-122, Feb-
ruary, 1971.

"Immunologic reactions of humans to cephalosporins,"
by L. D. Petz. POSTGRAD MED J 47:64-69, February,
1971

CHANCROID
"Ulcus molle in a woman," by H. R. Manuel, et al. NED
TIJDSCHR GENEESKD. 115:71, January 9, 1971.

CHILDREN
"Sexually transmitted infections in the schoolchild,"
by J. L. Fluker. MIDWIFE HEALTH VISIT. 6:91-96,
March, 1970.

"Urethritis in male children," by D. I. Williams, et
al. PROC R SOC MED. 64:133-134, February, 1971.

"Vaginal aspirate studies in children. An atraumatic
method," by V. J. Capraro, et al. OBSTET GYNECOL.
37:462-464, March, 1971.

CHLOROMYCETIN
"Chloromycetin failure in gonorrhea. A special case,"
by W Jadassohn. DERMATOLOGICA. 143:43-44, 1971.

COLLEGE STUDENTS AND VD
"Study of mycoplasma in university students with non-
gonococcal urethritis," by S. Sueltmann, et al.
HEALTH LAB SCI. 8:62-66, April, 1971.

COLPITIS

"Clinical and experimental results in colpitis therapy using Mysteclin," by H. Lohmeyer, et al. MED KLIN. 66:1278-1280, September 17, 1971.

"Lymecycline in Haemophilus vaginalis colpitis," by H. Fegeri, et al. WIEN MED WOCHENSCHR. 121:194-196, March 13, 1971.

"Thrush colpitis," by G. K. Doring. DTSCH MED WOCHENSCHR. 96:358, February 19, 1971.

CONTRACEPTION AND CONTRACEPTIVES

"The condom," by K. Flegel. N ENGL J MED. 286:218-219, January 27, 1972.

"Effectiveness of condoms in preventing V.D.," by N. J. Fiumara. N ENGL J MED. 285:972, October 21, 1971.

"Influence of gestogenic contraceptive pills on vaginal candidosis," by R. D. Catterall BR J VENER DIS. 47:45-47, February, 1971

"Influence of oral contraception upon the occurence of Candida albicans in the vagina," by H. Thulin. NORD MED. 85:399-401, April 1, 1971.

"Is pill to blame for VD rise?" AM DRUGGIST. 163:38 plus, May 17, 1971.

"Screening tests for gonorrhea in clinics for contraceptive advice," by V. Starch, et al NORD MED. 86:1430-1432, December 2, 1971.

"Vaginal moniliasis during pregnancy and during intake of oral contraceptives," by W. Gruber, et al. WIEN MED WOCHENSCHR. 120:898-900, November 28, 1970.

CONTRACEPTION AND CONTRACEPTIVES

"Vaginal yeast growth and contraceptive practices," by W. N. Spellacy, et al. OBSTET GYNECOL. 38:343-349, September, 1971.

"Venereal diseases and modern contraception," by M. Vojta. CESK GYNEKOL. 36:60-61, February, 1971.

COPIAMYCIN
"Microbiological study of copiamycin," by K. Seiga, et al. APPL MICROBIOL. 21:986-989, June, 1971.

CORTICOSTEROIDS
"Effect of corticosteroids on the Jarisch-Herxheimer reaction," by A. Luger, et al. WIEN KLIN WOCHEN-SCHR. 83:208-212, March 26, 1971.

DNA
"Atypical fluorescence in the fluorescent treponemal-antibody-absorption (FTA-ABS) test related to de-oxyribonucleic acid (DNA) antibodies," by S. J. Kraus, et al. J IMMUNOL. 106:1665-1669, June, 1971.

DENTISTRY
"Teaching of dermatologic and venereal diseases at the dental department," by B. M. Pashkov, et al. VESTN DERMATOL VENEROL. 45:68-72, November, 1971.

DETREOMYCIN
"Unsuccessful treatment of early symptomatic syphilis following oral administration of detreomycin, erythromycin and oxyterracin," by J. Lebioda, et al. PRZEGL LEK. 27:469-472, 1971.

DIAGNOSIS
"Better specimens from the female genital tract," by S. Selwyn, et al. BR MED J 4:170, October 16, 1971

94

DIAGNOSIS

"Diagnosis and treatment of venereal disease," by M.
Foster, Jr. POSTGRAD MED. 50:67-73, July, 1971.

"Errors in the diagnosis of acute and chronic non-
specific epididymitis," by B. S. Gekhman.
VOEN MED ZH. 1:43-45, January, 1971.

"Interactions of antilipoidal antibodies with yolk sac
antigens," by A. Lassus, et al. BR J VENER DIS.
47:169-172, June, 1971.

"A laboratory test is not a diagnosis," by N. J.
Fiumara. JAMA. 217:71, July 5, 1971.

"Technics of demonstration of IgM type antibodies in
congenital infections," by G. Dropsy, et al. ANN
BIOL CLIN. 29:67-73, 1971.

"Vaginal infections and infestations diagnosed by
cytology," by E. Gutiérrez Valverde, et al. GINECOL OB-
STET MEX. 30:619-625, December, 1971.

"Attempts to adapt Entamoeba histolytica to various
protozoan species in Diamond's TTY medium," by A.
Westphal, et al. Z TROPENMED PARASITOL. 22:149-
156, June, 1971.

DOXYCYCLINE
"Doxycycline treatment of nongonococcal urethritis
with special reference to T-strain mycoplasmas," by
A. Lassus, et al. BR J VENER DIS. 47:126-130,
April, 1971.

"Treatment of gonorrhea in women with doxycycline," by
J. Bartunek. MED WELT. 14:504-505, April 3, 1971.

"Treatment of gonorrhea with single oral doses. Results
obtained with doxycycline or rifampicin compared
with intramuscular pencillin," by E. P. Steenbergen.

DOXYCYCLINE

BR J VENER DIS. 47:111-113, April, 1971.

"Treatment of uncomplicated gonorrhea with a one time dose of doxycycline," by H. Hammar, et al. LAKARTID-NINGEN. 68:4278-4279, September 15, 1971.

"Treatment of uncomplicated gonorrhea with a single oral dose of doxycycline," by S. Liden. ACTA DERM VENEREOL. 51:221-224, 1971.

"Using one dose of doxycycline or penicillin to treat men with gonococcal urethritis," by S. R. Jones, et al   HSMHA HEALTH REP. 86:849-854, September, 1971.

DRUG ADDICTION
"Cutaneous and venereal diseases seen at a drug-oriented youth clinic," by R. N. Richards. ARCH DERMATOL. 104:438-440, October, 1971.

EDUCATION
"Overcoming teacher reluctancy toward VD education," by F. B. Benell. J SCH HEALTH. 40:483-486, November, 1970.

"Teaching about venereal diseases in medical schools," by C. J. Alarcon. BOL OF SANIT PANAM. 70:103-111, January, 1971.

"Teaching of dermatologic and venereal diseases at the dental department," by B. M. Pashkov, et al. VESTN DERMATOL VENEROL. 45:68-72, November, 1971.

"Venereal disease education," by M. Riggs. CALIF MED. 115:74-75, October, 1971.

"Venereal disease education program." ROCKY MT MED J. 68:28, December, 1971.

"Venereal disease education using a teaching question-

EDUCATION

naire," by R. M. Manuel, et al. CAN J PUBLIC HEALTH. 62:336-339, July - August, 1971.

EPIDIDYMITIS

"On the etiology of epididymitis," by L. H. Wolin. J UROL. 105:531-533, April, 1971.

ERYTHROMYCIN

"A case of failure in the treatment of early syphilis with erythromycin," by Z. Dratwinski. PRZEGL DERMATOL. 58:69-71, January - February, 1971.

"Unsuccessful treatment of early symptomatic syphilis following oral administration of detreomycin, erythromycin and oxyterracin," by J. Lebioda, et al. PRZEGL LEK. 27:469-472, 1971.

FERTILITY. INFERTILITY, AND STERILITY

"Mycoplasmas and fertility." DTSCH MED WOCHENSCHR. 96:223, January 29, 1971.

"Sterility in urogenital trichomoniasis," by J. Schmor. WIEN MED WOCHENSCHR. 120:808-812, November 14, 1970.

FLAGYL

See Metronidazole

GENTAMYCIN

"Results of the Nelson test during administration of gentamycin," by H. J. Heitmann, et al. Z HAUT GESCHLECHTSKR. 46:87-90, February 1, 1971.

GONORRHEA

"Antibiotic-resistant forms of gonorrheal infection," by F. V. Potapnev. VESTN DERMATOL VENEROL. 45:51-52, 1971.

"Atypical case of gonococcal bacteremia," by M. Jacobsen, et al. UGESKR LAEGER. 133:6-7, January 8, 1971.

"Atypical gonorrhoea." BR MED J. 3:322, August 7, 1971.

"Atypical gonorrhoea," by J. Vahrman. BR MED J. 3: 579-580, September 4, 1971.

"Bicillin-6 therapy of gonorrhea in men," by V. E. Grigoriev, et al. VESTN DERMATOL VENEROL. 45:74-77, January, 1971.

"Clinical picture of combined gonorrheal-trichomonad urethritis," by I. I. Mavrov, et al. VESTN DERMATOL VENEROL. 45:84-86, June, 1971.

"Current aspects of gonococcal disease," by L. Rouques. PRESSE MED. 7:1077, May 8, 1971.

"Current aspects of gonorrhea. Statistical study apropos of 200 patients," by P. Amblard, et al. LYON MED. 225:644, April 11, 1971.

"The current course of female gonorrhea," by J. Bartunek. Z HAUT GESCHLECHTSKR. 46:91-93, February 1, 1971.

"Desoxyribonuclease in Neisseria gonorrhoeae," by U. Berger. NATURWISSENSCHAFTEN. 58:63, January, 1971.

"Disseminated gonococcal infection," by K. K. Holmes, et al. ANN INTERN MED. 74:979-993, June, 1971.

"Epidemiological situation of lues and gonorrhea," by D. Petzoldt. MED KLIN. 66:335-338, March 5, 1971.

"Epidemiology of 25,294 reported gonorrhea cases," by G. R. Najem, et al. J OKLA STATE MED ASSOC. 64: 235-240, June, 1971.

"Gonorrhoea," by W. K. Bernfeld. NURS TIMES. 67:382-

383, April 1, 1971.

"Gonorrhea," by G. J. Pazin, et al. AM FAM PHYSICIAN.
3:124-137, June, 1971.

"Gonorrhea and gynecological examination during a
health survey," by K. Lindholm, et al. LAKARTID-
NINGEN. 68:4263-4264, September 15, 1971.

"Gonorrhea and tonsillitis following genito-oral contact," by L. Hellgren. LAKARTIDNINGEN. 68:569-
571, February 3, 1971.

"Gonorrhea epidemic." NEWSWEEK. 77:54, April 26, 1971.

"Gonorrhea in women," by M. Hart. JAMA. 216:1609-1611,
June 7, 1971.

"Gonorrhea in women," by C. S. Nicol. GYNAEKOL RUNDSCH.
10:182-189, 1970.

"Gonorrhea in women: treatment with sulfamethoxazole
and trimethoprim," by C. B. Schofield, et al. J
INFECT DIS. 124:533-538, December, 1971.

"Gonorrhea problems," by S. A. Kvorning. UGESKR
LAEGER. 133:1249-1252, July 2, 1971.

"The gonorrhea situation today," by H. Hansson. LAK-
ARTINDNINGEN. 68:4239-4241, September 15, 1971.

"Improved tracing of contacts of heterosexual men with
gonorrhoea. Relationship of altered female to male
ratios," by E. M. Dunlop, et al. BR J VENER DIS.
47:192-195, June, 1971.

"The prostate as a reservoir for gonococci," by D.
Danielsson, et al. LAKARTIDNINGEN. 68:4267, September 15, 1971.

GONORRHEA

"Record of a case of gonorrhea." INFIRM FR. 123:33, March, 1971.

"Syphilis and gonorrhea at the Munich University dermatological hospital 1959 - 1969," by D. Petzolt, et al. HAUTARZT. 22:253-257, June, 1971.

"Transfer of gonococcal urethritis from man to chimpanzee. An animal model for gonorrhea," by C. T. Lucas, et al. JAMA. 216:1612-1614, June 7, 1971.

"Transmission possibilities of gonorrhea?" by H. Gotz. MUNCH MED WOCHENSCHR. 113:742-743, May 7, 1971.

"VD: Gonorrhea incidence put at 2 million annually in U. S." HOSP PRACT. 6:27 plus, June, 1971.

"Venereal disease. Women, the unwitting carriers of gonorrhea," by P. E. Lenz. AM J NURS. 71:716-719, April, 1971.

"Virulence factors in gonococci." DTSCH MED WOCHENSCHR. 96:137, January 15, 1971.

GONORRHEA: ANO-RECTAL

"Anal soft chancre and concomitant gonorrhea," by J. Rivoire. BULL SOC FR DERMATOL SYPHILIGR. 78:203, 1971.

"Rectal gonorrhea in women," by K. Odegaard, et al. TIDSSKR NOR LAEGEFOREN. 91:1474-1476, July 10, 1971.

"Symptomatic anorectal gonorrhea in an adolescent female," by W. T. Speck, et al. AM J DIS CHILD. 122:438-439, November, 1971.

"Trimethoprim-sulphamethoxazole (Septrin) in the treatment of rectal gonorrhoea," by M. A. Waugh. BR J VENER DIS. 47:34-35, February, 1971.

GONORRHEA: ARTHRITIC

"Gonococcal arthritis. A survey of 54 cases," by C.
L. Cooke, et al. JAMA. 217:204-205, July 12, 1971.

"The gonococcal arthritis-dermatitis syndrome," by K.
K. Holmes, et al. ANN INTERN MED. 75:470-471,
September, 1971.

"Gonococcal arthritis in two patients with active
lupus erythematosus. A diagnostic problem," by J.
S. Edelen, et al. ARTHRITIS RHEUM. 14:557-559,
September - October, 1971.

"Gonococcal pharyngitis and arthritis," by F. LaLuna,
et al. ANN INTERN MED. 75:649, October, 1971.

"Gonococcal sepsis and arthritis." CALIF MED. 114:
18-25, January, 1971.

"Recovery of Neisseria gonorrhoeae from 'Sterile'
synovial fluid in gonococcal arthritis," by K. K.
Holmes, et al. N ENGL J MED. 284:318-320, February
11, 1971.

GONORRHEA: CEREBRO-SPINAL
"Gonococcal meningitis," by H. L. Taubin, et al. N
ENGL J MED. 285:504-505, August 26, 1971.

GONORRHEA: CHILDREN
"Gonococcal infections in prepubertal children," by V.
F. Burry, et al. MO MED. 68:691-692, September,
1971.

"Gonococcal vulvovaginitis and possible peritonitis in
prepubertal girls," by V. F. Burry. AM J DIS CHILD.
121:536-537, June, 1971.

"Gonorrhea in children," by A. Mark, et al. LAKARTID-
NINGEN. 68:4265-4266, September 15, 1971.

GONORRHEA: CHILDREN

"Nonvenereal transmission of gonococcal infections to children," by W. B. Shore, et al. J PEDIATR. 79: 661-663, October, 1971.

GONORRHEA: COMPLICATIONS
"Gonococcal sepsis," by J. Barr, et al. LAKARTIDNINGEN. 68:4255-4260, September 15, 1971.

"Gonococcal sepsis and arthritis." CALIF MED. 114:18-25, January, 1971.

"Gonorrheal-trichomonad urethritis in men," by A. I. Lopatin, et al. VESTN DERMATOL VENEROL. 45:53-56, July, 1971.

"Isolated affection of paraurethral ducts by gonorrheal infection," by F. V. Potapnev, et al. VESTN DERMATOL VENEROL. 45:83-84, June, 1971.

"Septic gonococcal dermatitis." BR MED J. 1:472-473, February 27, 1971.

"Septic gonococcal dermatitis," by J. Barr, et al. BR MED J. 1:482-485, February 27, 1971.

GONORRHEA: DIAGNOSIS
"An automated complement fixation procedure for detecting antibody to N. gonorrhoeae," by W. L. Peacock, Jr. HSMHA HEALTH REP. 86:706-710, August, 1971.

"A chemically definable enricher of culture media for Neisseria gonorrhoeae," by L. Posposil. CESK DERMATOL. 46:23-25, February, 1971.

"A comparative study of the laboratory diagnosis of gonorrhea," by J. R. Hodges, et al. HEALTH LAB SCI. 8:17-20, January, 1971.

"Demonstration of neisseria gonorrhoeae in prostatic

fluid after treatment of uncomplicated gonorrhoeal urethritis," by D. Danielsson, et al. ACTA DERM VENEREOL. 51:73-76, 1971.

"Determination of antibodies against Neisseria gonorrhoeae in gonorrhea patients," by E. Pulchartova, et al. CESK EPIDEMIOL MIKROBIOL IMUNOL. 20: 270-276, September, 1971.

"Diagnosis of gonorrhea," by J. Meyer-Rohn. Z ALLGE-MEINMED. 47:883-886, June 20, 1971.

"Diagnosis of gonorrhea with laboratory-technical methods, including the specific immunofluorescence test (FAT-Fluorescence Antibody Technic). II. Preparation of immune serums against Neisseria gonorrhoeae and studies on sensitization and specificity after labelling," by J. Mohr, et al. DTSCH GESUNDHEITSW. 26: 1758-1761, September 9, 1971.

"Direct and delayed methods of immunofluorescent diagnosis of gonorrhoea in women," by R. N. Thin, et al. BR J VENER DIS. 47:27-30, February, 1971.

"Evaluation of the gonococcal complement-fixation test," by C. S. Ratnatunga. BR J VENER DIS. 47:279-288, August, 1971.

"Experience with the diagnosis and treatment of gonorrhea in women," by V. Palous, et al. CESK DERMATOL. 46:256-261, December, 1971.

"Fluorescence method for determination of gonococci in venereologic practice," by H. Medebach. Z HAUT GES-CHLECHTSKR. 46:159-162, March 1, 1971.

"Gonorrhea diagnosis. Laboratory diagnostic point of view," by D. Danielsson. LAKARTIDNINGEN. 68:4242-4250, September 15, 1971.

"Gonorrhea masked by acne vulgaris treatment," by T.
A. Cortese, Jr.   JAMA.   216:330-331, April 12, 1971.

"Gonorrhea today: problems of diagnosis, management,
treatment," by R. C. Reznichek, et al.   CALIF MED.
115:32-38, August, 1971.

"Human serum antibodies reacting with endotoxin from
Neisseria gonorrhoeae," by J. A. Maeland, et al.
BR J VENER DIS.   47:269-272, August, 1971.

"Immunological reactivity of patients with gonorrhea,"
by L. D. Butovetskii, et al.   VESTN DERMATOL VENEROL.
45:56-59, 1971.

"The importance of cultural identification of Neisseria
gonorrhoeae for the diagnosis of problematic clinical
cases," by E. Friedrich, et al.   DTSCH GESUNDHEITSW.
26:401-404, February 25, 1971.

"Importance of gonococcal cultures and determination
of oxidase activity in the diagnosis of gonorrhea,"
by B. Raszeja-Kotelba, et al.   POL TYG LEK.   26:417-
419, March 22, 1971.

"Isovitalex--a chemically definable enricher of culture
media for Neisseria gonorrhoeae," by L. Pospisil.
CESK DERMATOL.   46:23-25, February, 1971.

"Microflocculation assay for gonococcal antibody," by
G. Reising.   APPL MICROBIOL.   21:852-853, May, 1971.

"Microscopy in the diagnosis of gonorrhea," by O. I.
Haavelsrud, et al.   TIDSSKR NOR LAEGEFOREN.   91:
1476-1477, July 10, 1971.

"Morphologic and histochemical changes in the mucosa
of the urogenital tract in gonorrhea, trichomonas
and candidiasis," by V. G. Bilik, et al.   VESTN

DERMATOL VENEROL. 45:50-53, May, 1971.

"Neisseria gonorrhoeae. 2. Colony variation," by A. Reyn, et al. ACTA PATHOL MICROBIOL. 79:435-436, 1971.

"Neisseria gonorrhoeae. 3. Demonstration of presumed appendages to cells from different colony types," by A. E. Jephcott, et al. ACTA PATHOL MICROBIOL SCAND. 79:437-439, 1971.

"The occurrence of oxidase-positive non-gonococcal strains on Thayer-Martin selective media used in the laboratory diagnostic of N. gonorrhoeae," by E. Geizer. ZENTRALBL BAKTERIOL. 214:75-78, 1970.

"On the antibiotic sensitivity of strains of Neisseria gonorrhoeae," by M. Peter, et al. MICROBIOL PARAZI-TOL EPIDEMIOL. 16:153-157, March - April, 1971.

"Present trends in the laboratory diagnosis of N. gonorrhoeae," by R. M. Breen. MED ANN DC. 40: 638-639, October, 1971.

"The preservation of gonococci in liquid nitrogen," by M. E. Ward, et al. J CLIN PATHOL. 24:122-123, March, 1971.

"Recommendations on the diagnosis of gonorrhea," by A. H. Rudolph, et al. JAMA. 218:448, October 18, 1971.

"Recovery of Neisseria gonorrhoeae from 'Sterile' synovial fluid in gonococcal arthritis," by K. K. Holmes, et al. N ENGL J MED. 284:318-320, February 11, 1971.

"Resurgence of gonorrhea and its diagnosis by the gonoreaction," by E. Russo. REV BRAS MED. 28:99-

103, March, 1971.

"Screening females for asymptomatic gonorrhea infection," by A. H. Pedersen, et al. NORTHWEST MED. 70:255-261, April, 1971.

"Screening tests for gonorrhea in clinics for contraceptive advice," by V. Starck, et al. NORD MED. 86:1430-1432, December 2, 1971.

"Sensitivity and reproducibility of Thayer-Martin culture medium in diagnosing gonorrhea in women," by J. G. Caldwell, et al. AM J OBSTET GYNECOL. 109:463-468, February 1, 1971.

"Serologic detection of gonorrhea," by B. B. Diena. ANN INTERN MED. 75:135, July, 1971.

"Solid non-agar egg medium for culture of Neisseria," by M. Pekowski, et al. POL TYG LEK. 26:988-990, June 28, 1971.

"Transgrow, a medium for transport and growth of Neisseria gonorrhoeae and Neisseria meningitidis," by J. E. Martin, et al. HSMHA HEALTH REP. 86:30-33, January, 1971.

"Trimethoprim for the prevention of overgrowth by swarming Proteus in the cultivation of gonococci," by K. Odegaard. ACTA PATHOL MICROBIOL SCAND. 79:545-548, 1971.

"Use of transport media in the cultural diagnosis of gonorrhea," by M. V. Iatsukha. VESTN DERMATOL VENEI OL. 45:58-61, November, 1971.

"Value of vaginal and rectal cultures in the diagnosis of gonorrhoea. With special reference to areas with limited medical facilities," by G. A. Olsen. BR J

GONORRHEA: DIAGNOSIS

VENER DIS. 47:102-106, April, 1971.

GONORRHEA: HEPATIC
"Acute gonococcal perihepatitis (Fitz-Hugh- Curtis
syndrome). An acute, right-side "pleuritic-peritonitic" upper abdominal pain syndrome in Adnexitis
gonorrhoica: diagnosis by laparoscopy," by R.
Amman, et al. DTSCH MED WOCHENSCHR. 96:1515-1519,
September 24, 1971.

GONORRHEA: NASO-PHARYNEGEAL
"Gonococcal pharyngitis and arthritis," by F. LaLuna,
et al. ANN INTERN MED. 75:649, October, 1971.

"Gonococcal tonsillar infections," by A. Bro-Jorgensen,
et al. BR MED J. 4:660-661, December 11, 1971.

"Gonococcal tonsillitis," by Y. Iqbal. BR J VENER DIS.
47:144-145, April, 1971.

"Gonorrhea and tonsillitis following genito-oral contact," by L. Hellgren. LAKARTIDNINGEN. 68:569-
571, February 3, 1971.

GONORRHEA: NEONATAL
"Diagnosis of gonorrheal infection by culture of the
external ear canal in the newborn," by J. W. Scanlon.
CLIN PEDIATR. 10:528-529, September, 1971.

"Gonococcal ophthalmia neonatorum despite treatment
with antibacterial eye-drops," by C. B. Schofield,
et al. BR MED J. 1:257-259, January 30, 1971.

GONORRHEA: OCCURRENCE
"Gonorrhoea in the family," by J. K. Oates. BR MED J.
3:580, September 4, 1971.

"Gonorrhea in a female out-patient-material," by P. A.
Mardh, et al. LAKARTIDNINGEN. 68:4261-4262, Septem-

ber 15, 1971.

"Incidence of gonorrhoea," by W. F. Felton. BR MED J.
4:683, December 11, 1971.

"Partial epidemiological analysis of gonorrhea cases
in a single Prague district," by K. Kopecky, et al.
CESK EPIDEMIOL MIKROBIOL IMUNOL. 20:195-202, July,
1971.

"Seasonality of gonorrhea in the United States," by
C. E. Cornelius, III. HSMHA HEALTH REP. 86:157-
160, February, 1971.

"Trends and status of gonorrhea in the United States,"
by W. J. Brown. INFECT DIS. 123:682-688, June, 197

GONORRHEA: OPHTHALMIC
"Gonorrheal conjunctivitis," by R. W. Thatcher, et al.
JAMA. 215:1494-1495, March 1, 1971.

"Prophylaxis of gonococcal ophthalmia." MED LETT DRUGS
THER. 12:38-39, May 1, 1970.

GONORRHEA: PENILE
"Case of gonnorrheic inflammation of the prepuce with
negative findings on gonococci in the urethra," by
A. Wierer, et al. CESK DERMATOL. 46:253-255, Decem
ber, 1971.

"Drug hits VD-related eye disease." AM DRUGGIST. 163:
34, June 28, 1971.

"Gonococcal tysonitis without urethritis after prophylactic post-coital urination," by J. A. Burgess.
BR J VENER DIS. 47:40-41, February, 1971.

"Primary gonorrheal abscess of the penile skin," by Z.
Ruszczak, et al. PRZEGL DERMATOL. 58:627-629,

GONORRHEA: PENILE

September - October, 1971.

GONORRHEA: PREVENTION AND CONTROL
"The current status of gonorrhoea control," by R. R.
Willcox. BR J CLIN PRACT. 25:215-222, May, 1971.

"The gonorrhea problem: action planning," by R. Grubb,
et al. LAKARTIDNINGEN. 68:4285-4288, September 15,
1971.

"The St. Claire County gonorrhea study: private and
public health resources combine in an effort to
control gonorrhea," by R. E. Rowe, et al. MICH MED.
70:317-318, April, 1971.

"Survey of gonorrhoea practices in Great Britain," by British Cooperative Clinical Group." BR J VENER DIS.
47:17-26, February, 1971.

"Treatment and prevention of syphilis and gonorrhea."
MED LETT DRUGS THER. 13:85-87, October, 1971.

"Venereal diseases as a problem of national and international health. Problems of control of gonorrhea,"
by S. A. Campos. SALUD PUBLICA MEX. 13:41-52,
January - February, 1971.

GONORRHEA: SERVICEMEN
"Army treatment of gonorrhea," by J. B. Grossman. ANN
INTERN MED. 75:135-136, July, 1971.

GONORRHEA: TREATMENT
"APP treats gonorrhea." AM DRUGGIST. 163:46, May 3,
1971.

"Antibodies to gonococcal lipopolysaccharides in patients
with gonorrhoea," by M. E. Ward, et al. J MED MICRO-
BIOL. 4:2-3, May, 1971.

"Blood penicillin levels in patients with gonorrhea treated according to various therapeutic schedules," by J. Bowszyc, et al. PRZEGL DERMATOL. 58:595-599, September - October, 1971.

"Chloromycetin failure in gonorrhea. A special case," by W. Jadassohn. DERMATOLOGICA. 143:43-44, 1971.

"Choice of penicillins for gonorrhoea." BR MED J. 2:485, May 29, 1971.

"Clinical trials with ampicillin in the treatment of gonorrheal urethritis in males," by S. Arap. HOSPITAL (Rio de Janeiro). 77:1173-1177, April, 1970.

"The current state of treatment of gonorrhoea with reference to decreased penicillin sensitivity of Neisseria gonorrhoeae," by J. Mayer-Rohn. BR J VENER DIS. 47:379, October, 1971.

"Current therapy of gonorrhea." JAMA. 218:714-717, November 1, 1971.

"Effect of double dose of aqueous procaine pencillin to treat gonorrhea in men," by M. Nelson. HSMHA HEALTH REP. 86:285-288, March, 1971.

"Epidemiology of gonococci with decreased sensitivity to penicillin in Malmo, South Sweden," by H. Moller. ACTA DERM VENEREOL. 51:77-80, 1971.

"An evaluation of bovine albumin and sodium glutamate in the lyophilization of Neisseria gonorrhoeae," by T. L. Klassen. CAN J MED TECHNOL. 33:147-154, August, 1971.

"Evaluation of treatment of gonorrhea in males with single doses of minocycline," by W. T. Tyson, Jr., et al. J TENN MED ASSOC. 64:773-777, September,

1971.

"Evolution of the sensitivity of the gonococcus to antibiotics. 3," by G. Niel, et al. PATHOL BIOL. 19:53-64, January, 1971.

"Hetacillin in single dose in the treatment of gonorrhea," by J. M. Barros, et al. REV SAUDE PUBLICA. 5:47-50, June, 1971.

"Monomycin in treating gonorrhea in women," by E. N. Turanova, et al. VESTN DERMATOL VENEROL. 45:59-62, 1971.

"Neisseria gonorrhoeae in prostatic fluid after treatment of uncomplicated gonorrhoeal urethritis." ACTA DERM VENEROL. 51:73-76, 1971.

"Nifuratrone and gonorrhea," by E. B. Smith, et al. ANTIMICROB AGENTS CHEMOTHER. 10:267-269, 1970.

"One-capsule treatment of gonorrhea with minocycline," by H. Pariser, et al. ANTIMICROB AGENTS CHEMOTHER. 10:211-213, 1970.

"One-day oral ampicillin-treatment of gonorrhea in young adults," by L. H. Shapiro, et al. OBSTET GYNECOL. 37:414-418, March, 1971.

"Oral ampicillin in uncomplicated gonorrhoea. 3. Results of treatment in women with positive rectal culture," by G. Eriksson. ACTA DERM VENEREOL. 51: 305-310, 1971.

"Oral ampicillin in uncomplicated gonorrhoea. 4. Comparison of pharmacological and clinical results," by G. Eriksson. ACTA DERM VENEREOL. 51:467-475, 1971.

"Oral single-dose treatment of male and female gonorrhea with ampicillin alone and combined with probenecid," by A. Bro-Jorgensen, et al. UGESKR LAE-
GER. 133:1253-1256, July 2, 1971.

"PAM plus probenecid and procaine penicillin plus
probenecid in gonorrhoea," by A. L. Hilton. BR J
VENER DIS. 47:107-110, April, 1971.

"Present pattern of antibiotic sensitivity of gonococcal
strains isolated in Bombay," by J. M. Moses, et al.
BR J VENER DIS. 47:273-278, August, 1971.

"Re-appraising the effect on incubating syphilis of
treatment for gonorrhoea," by K. R. Woodcock. BR
J VENER DIS. 47:95-101, April, 1971.

"Results of treatment of gonorrhea with penicillin in
the light of clinical observations and laboratory
examinations," by J. Bowszye, et al. PRZEGL DERMA-
TOL. 58:715-721, November - December, 1971.

"Rifadin (rifampicin) in the treatment of gonorrhoea
in Uganda. A controlled trial," by O. P. Arya, et
al. BR J VENER DIS. 47:184-187, June, 1971.

"Sensitivity and appearance of resistance to rifampicin
in N. gonorrhoeae," by I. Juhlin, et al. ACTA
PATHOL MICROBIOL SCAND. 79:445, 1971.

"The sensitivity of gonococci to different antibiotics,"
by D. Danielsson. LAKARTIDNINGEN. 68:4273-4277,
September 15, 1971.

"Sensitivity to antibiotics of gonococcal strains isolated from sailors at Rotterdam," by A. Wols-Van der
Wielen. BR J VENER DIS. 47:190-191, June, 1971.

"A single-dose treatment of gonococcal urethritis with

rifampicin," by V. L. Ongom. BR J VENER DIS. 47: 188-189, June, 1971.

"Single-dose treatment of gonorrhoea with penicillin or thiamphenicol and its effect on T. pallidum in experimental syphilis," by D. Petzold. BR J VENER DIS. 47:380, October, 1971.

"Single oral dose ampicillin-probenecid treatment of gonorrhea in the male," by P. A. Kvale, et al. JAMA. 215:1449-1453, March 1, 1971.

"Therapy and therapy-control in uncomplicated gonorrhea," by H. Hansson, et al. LAKARTIDNINGEN. 68: 4268-4272, September 15, 1971.

"Therapy for incubating syphilis. Effectiveness of gonorrhea treatment," by A. L. Schroeter, et al. JAMA. 218:711-713, November 1, 1971.

"Therapy of gonorrhea with tetracycline," by J. Danda, et al. CESK DERMATOL. 46:1-6, February, 1971.

"Treatment of gonorrhea," by L. J. Lancaster. JAMA. 217:1106, August 23, 1971.

"Treatment of gonorrhea," by F. L. Roberts. JAMA. 218: 446, October 18, 1971.

"Treatment of gonorrhea in women with Doxycycline," by J. Bartunek. MED WELT. 14:504-505, April 3, 1971.

"Treatment of gonorrhea in young girls," by M. Loza-Tulimowska, et al. PRZEGL DERMATOL. 58:183-186, March - April, 1971.

"Treatment of gonorrhoea with aqueous benzyl penicillin plus probenecid," by A. M. Niordson, et al. ACTA DERM VENEREOL. 51:311-314, 1971.

113

"Treatment of gonorrhoea with single oral doses. Results obtained with doxycycline or rifampicin compared with intramuscular penicillin," by E. P. Van Steenbergen. BR J VENER DIS. 47:111-113, April, 1971.

"Treatment of gonorrhea with sulphamethoxazole-trimethoprim (Bactrim)," by H. Svindland. TIDSSKR NOR LAEGEFOREN. 91:1753-1755, August, 1971.

"Treatment of gonorrhoea with two oral doses of antibiotics. Trials of cephalexin and of triple tetracycline," by R. R. Willcox. BR J VENER DIS. 47: 31-33, February, 1971.

"Treatment of uncomplicated gonorrhea with a one time dose of doxycycline," by H. Hammar, et al. LAKARTIDNINGEN. 68:4278-4279, September 15, 1971.

"Treatment of uncomplicated gonorrhoea with a single oral dose of doxycycline," by S. Liden, et al. ACTA DERM VENEREOL. 51:221-224, 1971.

"A trial in treatment of gonorrhea with a sulphonamide with prolonged effect (sulfapherin)," by B. L. Jorgensen. UGESKR LAEGER. 133:1257-1258, July 2, 1971

"Trimethoprim-sulphamethoxazole in gonorrhoea," by S. Ullman, et al. ACTA DERM VENEREOL. 51:394-396, 1971.

"Uncomplicated gonorrhea treated with Trimethoprim and sulphamethoxazol," by B. L. Jorgensen, et al. UGESKI LAEGER. 133:1259-1260, July 2, 1971.

"Use of single doses of thiamphenicol in gonococcal urethritis," by V. Rodrigues, et al. REV BRAS MED. 28:288-290, June, 1971.

GONORRHEA: TREATMENT

"Using one dose of doxycycline or penicillin to treat
men with gonococcal urethritis," by S. R. Jones,
et al. HSMHA HEALTH REP. 86:849-854, September,
1971.

GONORRHEA: YOUTH
"Gonorrhea in the adolescent," by R. Sanders. J TENN
MED ASSOC. 64:1052-1054, December, 1971.

GRANULOMA INGUINALE
"A phenomenon resembling opsonic adherence shown by
disaggregated cells of the transmissible venereal
tumour of the dog," by D. Cohen, et al. BR J EXP
PATHOL. 52:447-451, October, 1971.

"Venereal granuloma," by O. Mattos, et al. REV BRAS
MED. 28:265, June, 1971.

HEART DISEASE AND VD
"Arthritis, vaginitis and cardiac murmur," by S. Jacobs.
J LA STATE MED SOC. 123:179-182, May, 1971.

"Can we prevent heart disease?" by L. Werko. ANN IN-
TERN MED. 74:278-288, February, 1971.

HERPES
"Genital herpes and cervical cancer," by P. Leinikki,
et al. DUODECIM. 87:181-183, 1971.

"Genital herpes and cervical cancer," by A. Singer.
BR MED J. 1:458, February 20, 1971.

"Genital herpes in two social groups," by W. E. Rawls,
et al. AM J OBSTET GYNECOL. 110:682-689, July 1,
1971.

"Genital herpes infection and non-specific urethritis,"
by S. Jeansson, et al. BR MED J. 3:247, July 24,
1971.

"Genital herpesvirus hominis type 2 infection: an experimental model in cebus monkeys," by A. J. Nahmias, et al. SCIENCE. 171:297-298, January 22, 1971.

"Genital herpesvirus hominis type 2 infection of monkeys," by W. T. London, et al. OBSTET GYNECOL. 37: 501-503, April, 1971.

"Herpes simplex: diagnosis and management," by A. P. Ulbrich. J AM OSTEOPATH ASSOC. 70:1196-1198, July, 1971.

"Herpes simplex infections on the genitalia," by S. Jeansson, et al. LAKARTIDNINGEN. 68:467-471, January 27, 1971.

"Herpesvirus antibody and carcinoma in situ of the cervix," by L. W. Catalano, Jr., et al. JAMA. 217:447-450, July 26, 1971.

"Management of pregnancy complicated by genital herpes virus infection," by M. S. Amstey. OBSTET GYNECOL. 37:515-520, April, 1971.

"Perinatal risk associated with maternal genital herpes simplex virus infection," by A. J. Nahmias, et al. AM J OBSTET GYNECOL. 110:825-837, July 15, 1971.

"Relationship of herpes simplex genital infection and carcinoma of the cervix: population studies," by Y. M. Centifanto, et al. AM J OBSTET GYNECOL. 110: 690-692, July 1, 1971.

"Sexual activity and cervical carcinoma," by H. J. Buchsbaum. J IOWA MED SOC. 61:559, September, 1971.

"Transport of herpes simplex virus in Stuart's medium," by P. Rodin, et al. BR J VENER DIS. 47:198-199,

HERPES

June, 1971.

HETACILLIN
"Hetacillin in single dose in the treatment of gonorrhea," by J. M. Barros, et al. REV SAUDE PUBLICA.
5:47-50, June, 1971.

HISTORY
"Attitudes of hospitals in London to venereal disease
in the 18th and 19th centuries," by M. A. Waugh.
BR J VENER DIS. 47:146-150, April, 1971.

"Dermatological and venereal diseases told about in
the Bible," by B. Bafverstedt. LAKARTIDNINGEN. 68:
3793-3802, August 18, 1971.

HYDROCORTISONE
"Administration of oxytetracycline hydrochloride with
hydrocortisone (Oxycort aerosol) in the treatment
of non-specific vaginitis," by A. Ostrzenski. POL
TYG LEK. 26:283-284, February 22, 1971.

LAWS AND LEGISLATION
"Decree of Presidium of the Russian Republic supreme
soviet no. 881, amending and supplementing the Russian
Republic criminal code and criminal procedure code."
CURRENT DIG SOVIET PR. 23:24, November 23, 1971.

"New Arizona legislation for treatment of minors with
V. D.," by S. Dandoy. ARIZ MED. 28:529-530, July,
1971.

"New legislation for treating minors with venereal disease," by S. Dandoy. ARIZ NURSE. 24:55, September -
October, 1971.

LEVORIN
"Pyrolysis-gas chromatography of polyene antifungal
antibiotics: the nature of candicidin, levorin, and

LEVORIN

trichomycin," by H. J. Burrows, et al. J CHROMA-
TOGR. 53:566-571, December 23, 1971.

"Treatment of candidal vulvovaginitis and urethritis
with 1 per cent alcohol-water solution of levorin,"
by I. I. Shkliar, et al. VESTN DERMATOL VENEROL. 45
81-84, February, 1971.

LUPUS ERYTHEMATOSUS

"Atypical FTA-ABS test fluorescence in lupus erythematosus," by F. Jennis. JAMA. 215:488-489, January 18, 1971.

"Atypical FTA-ABS test reaction. An initial clue in
the diagnosis of lupus erythematosus," by S. J.
Kraus, et al. ARCH DERMATOL. 104:260-261, September, 1971.

"Gonococcal arthritis in two patients with active lupus
erythematosus. A diagnostic problem," by J. S.
Edelen, et al. ARTHRITIS RHEUM. 14:557-559, September-October, 1971.

"Positive fluorescent treponemal antibody test in
systemic lupus erythematosus in childhood: report
of a case," by R. P. Lesser, et al. J PEDIATR. 79:
1006-1008, December, 1971.

LYMECYCLINE

"Lymecycline in Haemophilus vaginalis colpitis," by
H. Fegerl, et al. WIEN MED WOCHENSCHR. 121:195-
196, March 13, 1971.

LYMPHOGRANULOMA VENEREUM

"Antibodies binding the complement with antigens of

viruses of the ornithosis-psittacosis-lymphogranuloma venereum group and neorickettsiae in various
population groups and domestic animals," by C.
Frygin, et al. PRZEGL EPIDEMIOL. 25:55-62, 1971.

"Case report of student aviator with unusual psy-
chosomatic symptoms," by J. R. Anderson. AEROSP
MED. 42:1217-1218, November, 1971.

"Clinical and epidemiological study of Nicolas-Favre
disease in Bordeaux," by J. M. Tamisier, et al.
BORD MED. 4:739-742, March, 1971.

"Study of Chlamydiae in patients with lymphogranuloma
venereum and urethritis attending a venereal disease clinic," by R. N. Philip, et al. BR J VENER
DIS. 47:114-121, April, 1971.

"Treatment of early syphilis and venereal lymphogran-
ulomatosis with doxycyclines," by H. Hevia, et al.
REV MED CHIL. 99:402-405, June, 1971.

MENINGOCOCCI
"Carbohydrate fermentation patterns of Neisseria
meningitidis determined by a microtiter method,"
by J. A Davies, et al. APPL MICROBIOL. 21:1072-
1074, June, 1971.

"Meningococci in vaginitis," by J. E. Gregory, et al.
AM J DIS CHILD. 121:423, May, 1971.

"Meningococcus and gonococcus: never the Twain--well,
hardly ever," by H. A. Feldman. N ENGL J MED. 285:
518-520, August 26, 1971.

METHYLMERCADONE
"Detection of Trichomonas vaginalis in patients with
complaints of leukorrhea and the effects of treatment with methylmercadone at the Kurume University,"

METHYLMERCADONE

by S. Kato, et al. SANFUJINKA JISSAI. 20:884-889, August, 1971.

METRONIDAZOLE

"Metronidazole as a possible reason for difficulty in diagnosis of syphilis," by I. I. Il'in, et al. VESTN DERMATOL VENEROL. 45:74-76, February, 1971.

"Perspectives in the treatment of protozoal diseases resistant to metronidazole," by I. De Carneri. TRANS R SOC TROP MED HYG. 65:268-270, 1971.

"Strains of Trichomonas vaginalis resistant to metronidazole," by L. M. Korik. VESTN DERMATOL VENEROL 45:77-80, January, 1971.

"Treatment of trichomoniasis in the female with a 5-day course of metronidazole," by A. N. McClean. BR J VENER DIS. 47:36-37, February, 1971.

"Treatment of vaginal inflammation with metronidazole," by K. Suk, et al. ZENTRALBL GYNAEKOL. 93:1380-1383, October 2, 1971.

"Treatment of vaginal trichomoniasis with Takimetol tablets (methronidazole preparation)," by H. Ishikawa, et al. SANFUJINKA JISSAI. 20:99-103, January, 1971.

"Trichomoniasis in a closed community: efficacy of metronidazole," by E. E. Keighley. BR MED J. 1: 207-209, January 23, 1971.

MINOCYCLINE

"Evaluation of treatment of gonorrhea in males with single doses of minocycline," by W. T. Tyson, et al. J TENN MED ASSOC. 64:773-777, September, 1971.

"In vivo resistance to metronidazole induced on four

MINOCYCLINE

recently isolated strains of Trichomonas vaginalis,"
by I. De Carneri, et al. ARZNEIM FORSCH. 21:377-
381, March, 1971.

"One-capsule treatment of gonorrhea with minocycline,"
by H. Pariser, et al. ANTIMICROB AGENTS CHEMOTHER.
10:211-213, 1970.

MINOR VD AND INFECTIONS
"Perspectives in the treatment of protozoal diseases
resistant to metronidazole," by I. De Carneri.
TRANS R SOC TROP MED HYG. 65:268-270, 1971.

MONOMYCIN
"Monomycin in treating gonorrhea in women," by E. N.
Turanova, et al. VESTN DERMATOL VENEROL. 45:59-
62, 1971.

MYCOPLASMAS
"Antibiotics in mycoplasma media and the temporary
storage of specimens containing mycoplasmas of the
genital tract," by C. S. Goodwin, et al. J CLIN
PATHOL. 24:286-287, April, 1971.

"Bacteria, viruses, and mycoplasmas in acute pneumonia
in adults," by F. R. Fekety, et al. AM REV RESP
DIS. 104:499-507, October, 1971.

"Birth weight and genital mycoplasmas in pregnancy,"
by P. Braun, et al. N ENGL J MED. 284:167-171,
January 28, 1971.

"Doxycycline treatment of nongonococcal urethritis
with special reference to T-strain mycoplasmas," by
A. Lassus, et al. BR J VENER DIS. 47:126-130,
April, 1971.

"The effect of antibiotic therapy on mycoplasma in the
female genital tract. In vitro and in vivo studies

on the sensitivity of Mycoplasma hominis and T-Mycoplasmas to tetracyclines and other antibiotics, by L. Westrom, et al. ACTA OBSTET GYNECOL SCAND. 50:25-31, 1971.

"In vitro sensitivity of mycoplasmas isolated from various animals and sewage to antibiotics and nitrofurans," by M. Ogata, et al. J ANTIBIOT. 24: 443-451, July, 1971.

"Intravascular coagulation and acute renal failure in a child with mycoplasma infection," by I. M. Nilsso⟩ ACTA MED SCAND. 189:359-365, May, 1971.

"Isolation of L-form bacteria and mycoplasma in inflam matory urologic diseases," by A. E. Sukhodol'skaia, et al. VRACH DELO. 12:5, June, 1971.

"Mycoplasma and vaginal cytology," by P. A. Mardh, et al. ACTA CYTOL. 15:310-315, May - June, 1971.

"Mycoplasma hominis and postpartum febrile complicatio⟩ by H. J. Harwick, et al. OBSTET GYNECOL. 37:765-768, May, 1971.

"Mycoplasma pneumoniae pneumonia in Helsinki 1962-1970 Epidemic pattern and autoimmune manifestations," by E. Jansson, et al. SCAND J INFECT DIS. 3:51-54, 1971.

"Mycoplasmas and the evidence for their pathogenicity in man," by D. Taylor-Robinson. PROC R SOC MED. 64:31-33, January, 1971.

"Mycoplasmas and fertility." DTSCH MED WOCHENSCHR. 96:223, January 29, 1971.

"Role of mycoplasma infection in the genesis of spon-taneous abortion," by M. A. Bashmakova, et al. VOP

OKHR MATERIN DET. 16:67-70, February, 1971.

"Sensitivity of mycoplasma suipneumoniae to penicillin-G," by N. F. Friis. ACTA VET SCAND. 12:120-121, 1971.

"Studies on T-strain mycoplasmas in nongonococcal urethritis," by E. Jansson, et al. BR J VENER DIS. 47:122-125, April, 1971.

"Study of mycoplasma in university students with non-gonococcal urethritis," by S. Sueltmann, et al. HEALTH LAB SCI. 8:62-66, April, 1971.

"T-strains of mycoplasma and nongonococcal urethritis," by H. Haas, et al. BR J VENER DIS. 47:131-134, April, 1971.

"Tetracycline inhibition of Mycoplasma ribosomal protein synthesis," by C. C. Fraterrigo, et al. J ANTIBIOT. 24:185-188, March, 1971.

"Therapy of viral, mycoplasmal and rickettsial infections," by M. W. Rytel, et al. WIS MED J. 70:116-120, April, 1971.

"Venereologic importance of mycoplasmas," by A. Horvath, et al. ORV HETIL. 112:1820-1822, August 1, 1971.

"Yaws, Mycoplasma pneumoniae and cold agglutinins in New Guineans," by P. B. Booth. MED J AUST. 1:715, March 27, 1971.

"Yaws, Mycoplasma pneumoniae and cold agglutinins in New Guineans," by J. Kariks. MED J AUST. 1:85-87, January 9, 1971.

MYSTECLIN

"Clinical and experimental results in colpitis therapy using Mysteclin," by H. Lohmeyer, et al. MED KLIN. 66:1278-1280, September 17, 1971.

NEISSER, ALBERT
"Albert Neisser (1855-1916)," by H. Schwarz. INVEST UROL. 8:478-480, January, 1971.

NEONATAL
"Exploration of delayed cutaneous hypersensitivity to candidine in newborn and young infants," by R. Carron, et al. PEDIATRIE. 26:259-264, April - May 1971.

"Reports from the obstetrical clinic in Leipzig. Prevention of eye inflammation in the newborn," by Crede. AM J DIS CHILD. 121:3-4, January, 1971.

"Sequelae of neonatal inclusion conjunctivitis and associated disease in parents," by C. H. Mordhorst, et al. AM J OPHTHALMOL. 71:861-867, April, 1971.

"Silver nitrate and the eyes of the newborn. Crede's contribution to preventive medicine," by G. B. Forbes, et al. AM J DIS CHILD. 121:1-3, January, 1971.

NIFURATEL
"Action of Nifuratel on lower genital infections," by M. Fayette. J MED LYON. 52:1445-1451, November 5, 1971.

NIFURATRONE
"Nifuratrone and gonorrhea," by E. B. Smith, et al. ANTIMICROB AGENTS CHEMOTHER. 10:267-269, 1970.

NITRIMIDAZINE
"Detection of the antitrichomonal drug nitrimidazine (Naxogin) in urine," by G. D. Morrison, et al. BR

NITRIMIDAZINE

J VENER DIS. 47:38-39, February, 1971.

"Nitrimidazine in the treatment of Trichomonas vaginalis vaginitis," by L. Cohen. BR J VENER DIS. 47:177-178, June, 1971.

"Nitrimidazine in the treatment of trichomoniasis," by M. Moffett, et al. BR J VENER DIS. 47:173-176, June, 1971.

NURSING AND VD
"Has the nurse any responsibility in the control of venereal diseases in the Nigerian community?" by M. N. Obayan. NIGER NURSE. 2:17-18, July, 1970.

"The nurse and VD control," by H. E. Ferrari. CAN NURSE. 67:28-30, July, 1971.

"Return to nursing! Changes in dermatology," by N. Thorne. NURS MIRROR. 133:30-35, September 3, 1971.

NYSTATIN
"Effect of nystatin on mycelial transformation of Candida albicans cells in the human serum," by H. Buluk, et al. MED DOSW MIKROBIOL. 23:175-181, 1971.

"Vaginal candidiasis treated with nystatin containing globules," by T. Lakos. ORV HETIL. 112:1712-1714, July 18, 1971.

OCCURRENCE
"The international incidence of venereal disease," by T. Guthe, et al. R SOC HEALTH J. 91:122-133, May - June, 1971.

OPHTHALMOLOGY
"Historical review of oculogenital disease," by P. Thygeson. AM J OPHTHALMOL. 71:975-985, May, 1971.

125

OPROPHENON

"Antimicrobial properties of oprophenon," by M. M. Rotmistrov, et al. MIKROBIOL ZH. 33:117-119, 1971.

ORAL CAVITY
"Parasitic protozoa in the human oral cavity and their clinical importance," by F. A. Musaev. STOMATO-LOGIA. 50:60-62, May - June, 1971.

OXYTERRACINE
"Unsuccessful treatment of early symptomatic syphilis following oral administration of detreomycin, ery-thromycin and oxyterracin," by J. Lebioda, et al. PRZEGL LEK. 27:469-472, 1971.

OXYTETRACYCLINE
"Administration of oxytetracycline hydrochloride with hydrocortisone (Oxycort Aerosol) in the treatment of non-specific vaginitis," by A. Ostrzenski. POL TYG LEK. 26:283-284, February 22, 1971.

"Efficacy of prolonged regimes of oxytetracycline in the treatment of nongonococcal urethritis," by J. John. BR J VENER DIS. 47:266-268, August, 1971.

"Oxytetracycline-nystatin in the prevention of candidal vaginitis," by M. Silverman, et al. AM J OBSTET GYNECOL. 111:398-404, October 1, 1971.

"Trichomonas and oxytetracycline," by S. Szanto. BR MED J. 2:467, May 22, 1971.

PENICILLIN
"Blood level studies on the depot effect of clemizole-penicillin G in antiluetic therapy," by D. Kleinhans Z HAUT GESCHLECHTSKR. 46:359-365, June 1, 1971.

"Blood penicillin levels in patients with gonorrhea treated according to various therapeutic schedules," by J. Bowszyc, et al. PRZEGL DERMATOL. 58:595-599,

PENICILLIN

September - October, 1971.

"Clinical progression of ocular syphilis and neurosyphilis despite treatment with massive doses of
penicillin. Failure to demonstrate treponemes in
affected tissues," by C. N. Sowmini. BR J VENER
DIS. 47:348-355, October, 1971.

"Clinico-laboratory data on penicillin therapy of
patients with gonorrhea," by M. N. Varshavskaya,
et al. VESTN DERMATOL VENEROL. 45:53-56, 1971.

"Continuous penicillin therapy of patients with infectious syphilis," by M. P. Frishman, et al. VESTN
DERMATOL VENEROL. 44:52-57, September, 1970.

"Continuous treatment of early forms of syphilis with
penicillin and bicillin," by IuF Korolev. VOEN MED
ZH. 7:76-77, 1971.

"Drug hits VD-related eye disease." AM DRUGGIST. 163:
34, June 28, 1971.

"Dynamics of antibody subsidence in early symptomatic
syphilis treated with penicillin," by I. Klersnicka -
Itman, et al. PRZEGL DERMATOL. 58:699-707, November - December, 1971.

"Effect of double dose of aqueous procaine penicillin
to treat gonorrhea in men," by M. Nelson. HSMHA
HEALTH REP. 86:285-288, March, 1971.

"Effect of penicillin and bicillin-1 in experimental
syphilis in rabbits (experimental electron microscopic study)," by N. M. Ovchinnikov, et al. VESTN
DERMATOL VENEROL. 45:42-47, June, 1971.

"Epidemiology of gonococci with decreased sensitivity
to penicillin in Malmo, South Sweden," by H. Moller.

PENICILLIN

ACTA DERM VENEREOL. 51:77-80, 1971.

"In vitro antimicrobial activity of 6(D(-)-amino-p-hydroxyphenylacetamido) penicillanic acid, a new semisynthetic penicillin," by H. C. Neu, et al. ANTIMICROB AGENTS CHEMOTHER. 10:407-410, 1970.

"In vitro studies on the mechanism of penicillin and ampicillin drug reactions," by Z. H. Haddad, et al. INT ARCH ALLERGY APPL IMMUNOL. 41:72-78, 1971.

"PAM plus probenecid and procaine penicillin plus probenecid in gonorrhoea," by A. L. Hilton. BR J VENER DIS. 47:107-110, April, 1971.

"Penicillin 'fatigue'," by K. Naess. TIDSSKR NOR LAEGEFOREN. 91:665-666, March 30, 1971.

"Penicillin therapy in 44 cases of primary and secondary syphilis," by B. A. Smithurst. MED J AUST. 2:248-250, July 31, 1971.

"Persistence of T. pallidum and its significance in penicillin-treated seropositive late syphilis," by L. Yogeswari, et al. BR J VENER DIS. 47:339-347, October, 1971.

"Prophylactic treatment with penicillin in venereal diseases," by A. Luger. HAUTARZT. 22:135, March, 1971.

"Results of treatment of gonorrhea with penicillin in the light of clinical observations and laboratory examinations," by J. Bowszyc, et al. PRZEGL DERMATOL. 58:715-721, November - December, 1971.

"Sensitivity of Mycoplasma suipneumoniae to penicillin-G.," by N. F. Friis. ACTA VET SCAND. 12:120-121, 1971.

PENICILLIN

"Serum, lymph node and testicular concentrations of
penicillin in 31 healthy or syphilitic rabbits
treated with penicillin," by J. C. Pechere, et al.
PATHOL BIOL. 19:49-52, January, 1971.

"Single-dose treatment of gonorrhoea with penicillin
or thiamphenicol and its effect on T. pallidum in
experimental syphilis," by D. Petzold. BR J VENER
DIS. 47:380, October, 1971.

"Site of action of efficacy of antisyphilitic treatment
with penicillin. II. Problems of penicillin dosage," by A. Luger. HAUTARZT. 22:1-6, January, 1971.

"Treatment of gonorrhoea with aqueous benzyl penicillin
plus probenecid," by A. M. Niordson, et al. ACTA
DERM VENEREOL. 51:311-314, 1971.

"Using one dose of doxycycline or penicillin to treat
men with gonococcal urethritis," by S. R. Jones, et
al. HSMHA HEALTH REP. 86:849-854, September, 1971.

"Venereal disease. TLC with the penicillin," by R.
Mathews. AM J NURS. 71:720-723, April, 1971.

PIMAFUCIN
"Pimafucin--a polyvalent vaginal therapeutic agent,"
by U. Heynen. Z ALLGEMEINMED. 47:829-830, June 31,
1971.

"Prevention of vaginal Candida proliferation by the
use of Pimafucin vaginal tablets during metronidazole
treatment," by I. Alteras. BRUX MED. 51:501-503,
July, 1971.

PIMARICIN
"Experimental pathology of pathogenic fungi. Microscopic detectable pathological changes in Candida
albicans due to pimaricin," by H. Rieth. MYKOSEN.

129

PIMARICIN

14:47-48, January 1, 1971.

"Treatment of vaginitis of diverse etiology with
pimaricin," by F. Bianchi. MINERVA GINECOL. 23:
489-492, May 31, 1971.

PINTA
"Langerhans' cells in late pinta. Ultrastructural ob-
servations in one case," by H. A. Rodriguez, et al.
ARCH PATHOL. 91:302-306, April, 1971.

"Neuro-ophthalmological study of late yaws and pinta.
II. The Caracas project," by J. L. Smith, et al.
BR J VENER DIS. 47:226-251, August, 1971.

PREGNANCY
"Birth weight and genital mycoplasmas in pregnancy,"
by P. Braun, et al. N ENGL J MED. 284:167-171,
January 28, 1971.

"Corynebacterium vaginale vaginitis in pregnant women,"
by J. F. Lewis, et al. AM J CLIN PATHOL. 56:580-
583, November, 1971.

"Epidemiologic associations between vaginal candidiasis
in the pregnant woman and oral thrush in newborn
infants," by A. M. Dolgopol'skaia, et al. VOPR OKHR
MATERIN DET. 16:50-54, February, 1971.

"Intrauterine pregnancy and coexistent pelvic inflammatory disease," by A. A. Acosta, et al. OBSTET
GYNECOL. 37:282-285, February, 1971.

"Management of pregnancy complicated by genital herpes
virus infection," by M. S. Amstey. OBSTET GYNECOL.
37:515-520, April, 1971.

"Mycoplasma hominis and postpartum febrile complications
by H. J. Harwick, et al. OBSTET GYNECOL. 37:765-

768, May, 1971.

"Perinatal risk associated with maternal genital herpes simplex virus infection," by A. J. Nahmias, et al. AM J OBSTET GYNECOL. 110:825-837, July 15, 1971.

"Perinatal tips," by P. M. Zavell. MICH MED. 70:123-124, February, 1971.

"Role of myoplasma infection in the gensis of spontaneous abortion," by M. A. Bashmakova, et al. VOPR OKHR MATERIN DET. 16:67-70, February, 1971.

"Tetracycline in pregnancy?" by B. G. Newman. ANN INTERN MED. 75:648-649, October, 1971.

"Vaginal moniliasis during pregnancy and during intake of oral contraceptives," by W. Gruber, et al. WIEN MED WOCHENSCHR. 120:898-900, November 28, 1970.

PREVENTION AND CONTROL
"Achievements in the control of dermatologic and venereal diseases in Yamal (40th anniversary of the formation of the Yamal-Nenets National Region)," by N. A. Belonogova, et al. VESTN DERMATOL VENEROL. 45:61-63, June, 1971.

"Achievements in dermatovenereology in Georgia (1921-1971)," by L. T. Shetsiruli, et al. VESTN DERMATOL VENEROL. 45:72-76, November, 1971.

"'Blitz' proves effective public health tool," by C. F. Jacobs, et al. J LA STATE MED SOC. 123:417, September, 1971.

"Communities strike back," by W. F. Swartz. AMER J NURS. 71:724, April, 1971.

"Control of venereal diseases." LANCET. 2:807-808,

October 9, 1971.

"Control of venereal diseases in Petrograd, 1918-1919,"
by V. A. Bazanov. VESTN DERMATOL VENEROL. 45:65-
69, 1971.

"Gaps in venereology." BR MED J. 2:547, June 5, 1971.

"'Let's get VD'," by C. B. Kanterman. DENT STUD. 49:
20, May, 1971.

"Participation of the Department of Dermatologic and
Venereal Diseases of the Grodno Medical Institute
in the work of regional dermato-venereological net-
work," by L. I. Gokinaeva. VESTN DERMATOL VENEROL.
45:60-61, June, 1971.

"Prevention of communicable diseases in Mexico. V.
Pinta. Situation in Mexico in 1970," by G. Gosset-
Osuna. GAC MED MEX. 101:167-175, February, 1971.

"The prevention of venereal disease," by V. G. Cave.
J NATL MED ASSOC. January, 1971, p. 66-68.

"Progonasyl for VD prophylaxis?" by E. H. Braff.
CALIF MED. 115:75, October, 1971.

"The public health investigator's expanding role," by
T. W. Mathias. HSMHA HEALTH REP. 86:107-110,
February, 1971.

"Public health report." CALIF MED. 115:78-79, October,
1971.

"The reporting of venereal disease by physicians," by
R. H. Vanderhook. J INDIANA STATE MED ASSOC. 64:
1187-1188, November, 1971.

"Responsibility of the physician in the control of

venereal disease." NY STATE J MED. 71:1717, July 15, 1971.

"Social antivenereal activity of the Polish Eugenic Society in Warsaw (1916-1939). A contribution to the history of medical societies," by R. Zablotniak. POL MED J. 10:1024-1030, 1971.

"Some results and prospects of scientific research of the Department of Dermatologic and Venereal Diseases of the Tashkent Medical Institute," by A. A. Akovbian. VESTN DERMATOL VENEROL. 44:3-7, September, 1970.

"To fight VD." J PRACT NURS. 21:13, March, 1971.

"Today's values; how can we stop the spread of venereal disease?" by E. McConnell. FORECAST HOME ECON. 17: 30-31, November, 1971.

"Experience of work of the Chair of Skin and venereal Diseases in aiding public health organizations," by N. A. Torsuev, et al. VESTN DERMATOL VENEROL. 45:57-60, September, 1971.

PROBENECID

"Oral single-dose treatment of male and female gonorrhea with ampicillin alone and combined with probenecid," by A. Bro-Jorgensen, et al. UGESKR LAEGER. 133:1253-1256, July 2, 1971.

"PAM plus probenecid and procaine penicillin plus probenecid in gonorrhoea," by A. L. Hilton. BR J VENER DIS. 47:107-110, April, 1971.

"Single dose cures 96% of VD cases." AM DRUGGIST. 163: 62-63, June 14, 1971.

"Single oral dose ampicillin-probenecid treatment of

PROBENECID

gonorrhea in the male," by P. A. Kvale, et al. JAMA.
215:1449-1453, March 1, 1971.

"Treatment of gonorrhoea with aqueous benzyl penicillin
plus probenecid," by A. M. Niordson, et al. ACTA
DERM VENEREOL. 51:311-314, 1971.

PROGONASYL
"Progonasyl for VD prophylaxis?" by E. H. Braff, CALIF
MED. 115:75, October, 1971.

PROSTATITIS
"Treatment of prostatitis," by D. Volter. DTSCH MED
WOCHENSCHR. 96:1091-1093, June 18, 1971.

"A venereological view of the prostate gland," by L.
Molin. LAKARTIDNINGEN. 68:3500-3504, July 28, 1971.

PROSTITUTION
"Medical inspection of prostitutes in America in the
nineteenth century: the St. Louis experiment and
its sequel," by J. C. Burnham. BULL HIST MED. 45:
203-218, May - June, 1971.

PSYCHOLOGY, PERSONALITY AND VD
"Good personality breakdown in patients attending
venereal diseases clinics," by E. C. de Kite. BR J
VENER DIS. 47:135-141, April, 1971.

"Psychological aspects in venereology," by F. Novotny.
CESK DERMATOL. 46:77-82, April, 1971.

"Psychopathology in V. D. practice," by A. N. Boneff.
INDIAN J DERMATOL. 16:51-54, April, 1971.

"Psycho-social aspects of venereal diseases in teen-
agers," by I. Datt. INDIAN J DERMATOL. 16:27-35,
January, 1971.

PSYCHOLOGY, PERSONALITY AND VD

"Schizophrenic syndrome in congenital syphilis," by
O. Skalickova, et al. CESK PSYCHIATR. 67:260-
264, October, 1971.

"Sexual behaviour of male Pakistanis attending venereal
disease clinics in Great Britain," by A. S. Hossain.
SOC SCI MED. 5:227-241, June, 1971.

PYRIMIDINE
"Effect of pyrimidine derivatives on the formation of
anti-Candida immunity," by E. N. Bol'shakova. ZH
MIKROBIOL EPIDEMIOL IMMUNOBIOL. 48:59-61, February,
1971.

PYRITHIONE
"Study of the trichomonacidal properties of pyrithione
(sodium salt of 1-hydroxy-2 (1, H)-pyridinethione),"
by R. Cavier, et al. ANN PHARM FR. 28:211-214,
March, 1971.

PYROGENALE
"Late results of treating syphilis with bicillin-1,3,
4 and bicillin-3,4 in combination with pyrogenal,"
by T. V. Vasil'ev. VESTN DERMATOL VENEROL. 45:50-
58, January, 1971.

REACTIONS
"Apparent transient false-positive FTA-ABS test following small pox vaccination." J OKLA STATE MED ASSOC.
64:372, September, 1971.

"Drug allergy. I." BR MED J. 2:37-40, April 3, 1971.

"Drug allergy. II." BR MED J. 2:100-101, April 10,
1971.

"The reaction of the isoenzymes of transaldolase with
chlorodinitrobenzene," by O. Tsolas, et al. ARCH
BIOCHEM BIOPHYS. 143:516-525, April, 1971.

REACTIONS: AMPICILLIN

"Ampicillin rashes in glandular fever," by H. Pullen.
BR MED J. 2:653, June 12, 1971.

REACTIONS: JARISCH-HERXHEIMER
"Effect of corticosteroids on the Jarisch-Herxheimer
reaction," by A. Luger, et al. WIEN KLIN WOCHENSCHR.
83:208- 212, March 26, 1971.

"Physiologic changes during the Jarisch-Herxheimer reaction in early syphilis. A comparison with louse-
borne relapsing fever," by D. A. Warrell, et al.
AM J MED. 51:176-185, August, 1971.

"Rare cases of Herxheimer's reaction in a 1-month-old
infant with hemolytic jaundice in the course of
congenital syphilis," by K. Jaegermann. PRZEGL
EPIDEMIOL. 25:441-443, 1971.

REACTIONS: PENICILLIN
"Acute, hypersensitivity reaction to penicillin during
general anesthesia: a case report," by D. R. Cook,
et al. ANESTH ANALG. 50:152-155, January - February
1971.

"Anaphylactic reaction to oral penicillin," by J. P.
Geyman. CALIF MED. 114:87-89, May, 1971.

"Anaphylactic reaction after oral penicillin medication
by P. E. Waaler. TIDSSKR NOR LAEGEFOREN. 91:213-
214, January 30, 1971.

"Differing patterns of wheal and flare skin reactivity
in patients allergic to the penicillins," by R. G.
Van Dellen, et al. J ALLERGY. 47:230-236, April,
1971.

"The influence of penicillinase on hapten inhibitions
in vitro and in vivo in experimental penicillin
allergy," by D. Kraft, et al. Z IMMUNITAETSFORSCH

REACTIONS: PENICILLIN

ALLERG KLIN IMMUNOL. 141:265-273, 1971.

"Inhibitions with haptens in penicillin allergy," by
    H. P. Werner, et al. WIEN KLIN WOCHENSCHR. 83:
    194-196, March 19, 1971.

"Microangiopathic hemolysis and thrombocytopenia re-
    lated to penicillin drugs," by J. C. Parker, et al.
    ARCH INTERN MED. 127:474-477, March, 1971.

"The problem of penicillin allergy," by J. W. Smith.
    ARIZ MED. 28:305-307, April, 1971.

"Routine use of penicillin skin testing on an inpatient
    service," by N. F. Adkinson, Jr. N ENGL J MED.
    285:22-24, July 1, 1971.

"Skin tests in penicillin allergy," by H. Hellenbroich.
    HAUTARZT. 22:18-24, January, 1971.

"The usefulness of immediate skin tests to haptenes
    derived from penicillin. A study in patients with
    a history of previous adverse reactions to penicillin,"
    by M. J. Fellner, et al. ARCH DERMATOL. 103:371-
    374, April, 1971.

REITERS DISEASE
  See Syphilis

RIFAMPICIN
  "Rifadin (rifampicin) in the treatment of gonorrhoea
    in Uganda. A controlled trial," by O. P. Arya, et
    al. BR J VENER DIS. 47:184-187, June, 1971.

  "Sensitivity and appearance of resistance to rifampicin
    in N. gonorrhoeae," by I. Juhlin, et al. ACTA
    PATHOL MICROBIOL SCAND. 79:445, 1971.

  "A 'single dose' treatment of gonococcal urethritis

RIFAMPICIN

with rifampicin," by V. L. Ongom. BR J VENER DIS. 47:188-189, June, 1971.

"Treatment of gonorrhoea with single oral doses. Results obtained with doxycycline or rifampicin compared with intramuscular penicillin," by E. P. Van Steenbergen. BR J VENER DIS. 47:111-113, April, 1971.

SALPINGITIS
"Ampicillin in the treatment of gonorrheal salpingitis," by E. Hedberg, et al. LAKARTIDNINGEN. 68:335-340, January 20, 1971.

"Gonorrhea--salpingitis," by V. Falk. LAKARTIDNINGEN. 68:4250-4254, September 15, 1971.

SEROLOGY
"Application of the semi-automatic disposable tip pipette to routine serologic test," by P. K. Carter, et al. AM J MED TECHNOL. 37:87-89, March, 1971.

"Serological study in normal animals," by A. Utrilla. ACTAS DERMOSIFILIOGR. 61:1-12, January - February, 1970.

"Serology of venereal infections," by J. Meyer-Rohn. Z ALLGEMEINMED. 47:887-890, June 20, 1971.

SERVICEMEN
"A nationwide serum survey of Argentinian military recruits, 1965-1966. I. Description of sample and antibody patterns with arboviruses, polioviruses, respiratory viruses, tetanus and treponematosis," by A. S. Evans, et al. AM J EPIDEMIOL. 93:111-121, February, 1971.

"Sensitivity to antibiotics of gonococcal strains isolated from sailors at Rotterdam," by A. Wols-Van

SERVICEMEN

Der Wielen. BR J VENER DIS. 47:190-191, June, 1971.

SILVER NITRATE
"Silver nitrate and the eyes of the newborn. Crede's
contribution to preventive medicine," by G. B.
Forbes, et al. AM J DIS CHILD. 121:1-3, January,
1971.

SITUDICINE
"Trial of Situdicine in gynecologic therapy," by M.
Bruhat, et al. LYON MED. 225:773-775, April 25,
1971.

SOCIOLOGY AND BEHAVIOR
See also: Psychology, Personality and VD

"The economic repercussions of venereal diseases," by
A. E. Callin. BOL OF SANIT PANAM. 70:95-102, January, 1971.

"Living environment of Pakistani immigrants attending
venereal disease clinics in Britain," by A. S. Hossain. PUBLIC HEALTH. 85:123-131, March, 1971.

"Other people's disease." EMERGENCY MED. 3:126-127,
March, 1971.

"Sequelae of sexual freedom: the sexually transmitted
diseases," by C. S. Nicol. PROC R SOC MED. 64:
1108-1111, November, 1971.

"Socio-medical aspects of patients with venereal diseases," by N. Gustavsson. LAKARTIDNINGEN. 68:4280-
4284, September 15, 1971.

SULPHAMETHOXAZOLE
See Trimethoprim - Sulphamethoxazole

SULFAPHERIN

"A trial in treatment of gonorrhea with a sulphonamide with prolonged effect (sulfapherin)," by B. L. Jorgensen. UGESKR LAEGER. 133:1257-1258, July 2, 1971.

SYPHILIS

"Amino acid composition of treponemes," by C. W. Moss, et al. BR J VENER DIS. 47:165-168, June, 1971.

"Brucellosis and syphilis transmitted by transfusion," by A. Becerra-Garcia. GAC MED MEX. 101:699-701, June, 1971.

"Characteristics of current latent syphilis," by T. V. Vasil'ev, et al. VESTN DERMATOL VENEROL. 45:45-50, July, 1971.

"Chemistry of axial filaments of Treponema zuezerae," by M. A. Bharier, et al. J BACTERIOL. 150:422-429, January, 1971.

"Clinical and therapeutic aspects of syphilis," by H. Storck. PRAXIS. 60:412-419, March 30, 1971.

"Cryoblobulin and rheumatoid factor during primosecondary syphilis," by H. Perrot, et al. PRESSE MED. 7:1059-1060, May 8, 1971.

"Epidemiological situation of lues and gonorrhea," by D. Petzoldt. MED KLIN. 66:335-338, March 5, 1971.

"Epidemiology of syphilis," by H. Tsugami, et al. SAISHIN IGAKU. 26:1890-1896, October, 1971.

"Epidemy of soft chancres (9 cases)," by H. Thiers, et al. BULL SOC FR DERMATOL SYPHILIGR. 78:202, 1971.

"A ghost: soft chancre. Apropos of 2 recent cases," by D. Colomb, et al. LYON MED. 225:647-648, April

SYPHILIS

11, 1971.

"Horny syphilide," by C. N. Sowmini, et al. BR J
VENER DIS. 47:213-215, June, 1971.

"Reiter's disease," by J. J. De Blecourt. NED
TIJDSCHR BENEESKD. 115:97-100, January 16, 1971.

"Research on the treponematoses." WHO CHRON. 25:
112-116, March, 1971.

"Some urgent problems of current syphilidology," by
A. A. Studnitsin, et al. VESTN DERMATOL VENEROL.
45:3-9, July, 1971.

"Syphilis." CALIF MED. 115:47-60, August, 1971.

"Syphilis." CLIN SYMPOSIA. 23,3:3-32, 1971.

"Syphilis," by K. Mizuoka. NAIKA. 27:1256-1260,
June, 1971.

"Syphilis and gonorrhea at the Munich University dermatological hospital, 1959-1969," by D. Petzoldt, et
al. HAUTARZT. 22:253-257, June, 1971.

"Tertiary syphilis," by R. Degos, et al. BULL SOC FR
DERMATOL SYPHILIGR. 78:287-288, 1971.

SYPHILIS: AURAL
"Apropos of 2 cases of auricular syphilis," by E.
Poilpre, et al. REV OTONEUROOPHTALMOL. 43:136-
140, April, 1971.

SYPHILIS: CARDIOVASCULAR

"Aortic rupture secondary to a suprasigmoid syphilitic
gumma. Aortic insufficiency and fatal hemopericardium," by P. Louis, et al. COEUR MED INTERNE. 10:

313-321, April - June, 1971.

"A case of syphilitic aneurysm of the aortic sinus and aortic regurgitation," by S. Okawa, et al. JAP HEART J. 12:105-110, January, 1971.

"Linear calcification of the aorta," by M. C. Thorner. JAMA. 215:297, January 11, 1971.

"Luetic aneurysm of the descended aortic arch with neurologic complications (case report)," by Z. Novak, et al. NEUROPSIHIJATRIJA. 18:179-189, 1970.

"Luetic thoraco-lumbal aortic aneurysm with arrosion of the vertebral body," by I. Boldt, et al. FORT-SCHR GEB ROENTGENSTR NUKLEARMED. 114:846-849, June, 1971.

"Pathogenetic value of intracranial blood flow in a case of median cerebral artery occlusion associated with homolateral hemiplegia," by J. Sole-Lienas, et al. NEUROCHIRURGIA. 14:225-231, November, 1971.

"Syphilis of the aorta in the autopsy material of the Pathological Institute of the Medical Academy in Lubeck, in the years 1949-1968," by H. G. Gurich, et al. ZENTRALBL ALLG PATHOL. 114:499-504, 1971.

"Syphilitic aortic aneurysm," by J. A. Greenberg. N ENGL J MED. 284:394, February 18, 1971.

"Syphilitic aortitis in the aged," by P. Armand, et al. MARS MED. 108:455-458, 1971.

"Syphilitic ostial coronaritis. Analysis of 6 observations," by P. Michaud, et al. J CARDIOVASC SURG. 12:254-263, May - June, 1971.

SYPHILIS: CEREBROSPINAL

"Case of cerebral gumma of the left temporal lobe,"
by K. Kinoshita. BRAIN NERVE. 23:365-368, April,
1971.

"Clinical, immunochemical and serological studies of
dementia paralytica (GPI)," by H. Schmidt, et al.
INT ARCH ALLERGY APPL IMMUNOL. 40:851-860, 1971.

"Cranial lacunas in secondary syphilis," by P. Amblard, et al. BULL SOC FR DERMATOL SYPHILIGR. 78:
310-311, 1971.

"Cranial lacunar osteitis in secondary syphillis," by
G. Cabanel, et al. PRESSE MED. 79:1755-1756,
September 25, 1971.

SYPHILIS: CHILDREN
"Case of congenital neurosyphilis with a picture of
juevenile progressive paralysis," by W. Nyka.
NEUROPATOL POL. 9:353-357, October - December, 1971.

"A case of juvenile angina pectoris probably due to
congenital syphilis," by T. Kobayashi, et al. JAP
CIRC J. 35:221-226, February, 1971.

"Progressive syphilitic paresis in a 12-year-old girl,"
by Z. Goscinska, et al. PEDIATR POL. 46:369-371,
March, 1971.

"Spurious manifestations of cerebral tumor in the
course of hysterica reaction in a child with syphilitic encephalopathy," by A. Bratkowa. POL TYG
LEK. 26:217-218, July 8, 1971.

SYPHILIS: COMPLICATIONS
"A case of historical syphilis," by F. X. Carton, et
al. BULL SOC FR DERMATOL SYPHILIGR. 78:284-285,
1971.

"A case of mycosis fungoides (in lues latens sero-positiva) with radiographically detectable pulmonary granulomas," by H. Standau, et al. Z HAUT GES-CHLECHTSKR. 46:379-385, June 15, 1971.

"Cell-mediated immunity and lymphocyte transformation in syphilis," by G. M. Levene, et al. PROC R SOC MED. 64:426-428, April, 1971.

"A combination of primary syphilis and trichomonal balanoposthitis," by E. L. Fridman. VESTN DERMATOL VENEROL. 45:67-69, 1971.

"Lymphadenopathy in secondary syphilis," by D. R. Turner J PATHOL. 104:x, July, 1971.

"Nephrotic syndrome: a complication of secondary syphilis," by M. D. Hellier, et al. BR MED J. 4: 404-405, November 13, 1971.

"Sarcoid-like granulomas in secondary syphilis. A clinical and histopathologic study of five cases," by L. B. Kahn, et al. ARCH PATHOL. 92:334-337, November, 1971.

"Sarcoidal reaction of the skin in syphilis," by R. Singh, et al. BR J VENER DIS. 47:209-211, June, 1971.

"Secondary syphilis with chickenpox in an adult," by N. J. Fiumara, et al. BR J VENER DIS. 47:142-143, April, 1971.

"Witkop disease. Two 'favoid' cases due to syphilis," by P. S. Jain. BR J VENER DIS. 47:216-217, June, 1971.

"CBC done-no VDRL-results: two congenital syphilitics,"
by H. P. Hines, et al.   JAP J PHYSIOL.   67:309-310,
July, 1971.

"A case of juvenile angina pectoris probably due to
congenital syphilis," by T. Kobayashi, et al.   JAP
CIRC J.   35:221-226, February, 1971.

"Congenital syphilis."   ETHIOP MED J.   8:161-162,
October, 1970.

"Congenital syphilis," by N. O. Bwibo.   EAST AFR MED
J.   48:185-191, April, 1971.

"Congenital syphilis," by W. H. Eaglstein.   ARCH DERMA-
TOL.   103:524-526, May, 1971.

"Congenital syphilis," by T. C. Fleming, et al.   J BONE
JOINT SURG.   53:1648-1651, December, 1971.

"Congenital syphilis," by Z. Sternadel.   PIELEG POLOZNA.
7:10-11, July, 1970.

"Congenital syphilis and its prevention," by D. L.
Pereldik.   FELDSHER AKUSH.   36:26-29, April, 1971.

"Congenital syphilis in Addis Ababa," by Y. Larsson,
et al.   ETHIOP MED J.   8:163-172, October, 1970.

"Congenital syphilis: a nonvenereal disease," by J.
G. Caldwell.   AM J NURS.   71:1768-1772, September,
1971.

"Congenital syphilis: resurgence of an old problem,"
by R. H. Wilkinson, et al.   PEDIATRICS.   47:27-
30, January, 1971.

"Early congenital bone syphilis: various clinical and
radiological aspects," by A. Fazzi, et al.   REV PAUL

SYPHILIS: CONGENITAL

MED. 77:73-76, March, 1971.

"Hutchinson's teeth and early treatment of congenital
syphilis," by W. K. Bernfeld. BR J VENER DIS. 47:
54-56, February, 1971.

"Infantile congenital syphilis. Presenting with bilateral orchitis," by R. Singh, et al. BR J VENER
DIS. 47:206-208, June, 1971.

"Schizophrenic syndrome in congenital syphilis," by O.
Skalickova, et al. CESK PSYCHIATR. 67:260-264,
October, 1971.

"Study of 2 cases of congenital syphilitic hepatitis
with biopsy," by G. Lepercq, et al. ANN MED INTERNE
122:633-638, May, 1971.

SYPHILIS: CUTANEOUS
"2 rare cases of secondary syphilis," by M. F. Roitburd
VESTN DERMATOL VENEROL. 44:76-79, November, 1970.

SYPHILIS: DIAGNOSIS
See also: Tests
            Syphillis: Serology and Serodiagnosis

"Acquired syphilis--drugs and blood tests," by W. J.
Brown. AMER J NURS. 71:713-715, April, 1971.

"The Automated reagin Test (ART) for syphilis in a
public health laboratory," by B. S. West, et al.
HEALTH LAB SCI. 8:220-224, October, 1971.

"Automated reagin test for syphilis in a multichannel
blood grouping machine," by A. L. Schroeter, et al.
AM J CLIN PATHOL. 56:43-49, July, 1971.

"Automatic indirect immunofluorescence applied to
syphilis serology (AFTA)," by S. S. Kasatiya, et al.

CAN J PUBLIC HEALTH. 62:166-168, March - April, 1971.

"Clinical progression of ocular syphilis and neuro-syphilis despite treatment with massive doses of penicillin. Failure to demonstrate treponemes in affected tissues," by C. N. Sowmini. BR J VENER DIS. 47:348-355, October, 1971.

"Clinico-radiologic manifestations of gummatous syphilis involving the soft tissues," by P. D. Khazov. VESTN DERMATOL VENEROL. 45:85-87, February, 1971.

"Comparative study of serologic reactions for the diagnosis of syphilis," by A. Sirena, et al. PRENSA MED ARGENT. 58:1691-1695, October 22, 1971.

"Comparison of direct and indirect fluorescent antibody methods for staining Treponema pallidum," by F. J. Elsas. BR J VENER DIS. 47:255-258, August, 1971.

"Complement-fixing antibodies to Bedsonia in Reiter's syndrome, TRIC agent infection, and control groups," by J. Schachter. AM J OPHTHALMOL. 71:857-860, April, 1971.

"Diagnosis and treatment of syphilis," by P. F. Sparling. N ENGL J MED. 284:642-653, March 25, 1971.

"The diagnosis of infectious syphilis," by F. B. Desmond. NZ MED J. 73:135-138, March, 1971.

"Eletron microscopic observations on the structure of Treponema zuelzerae and its axial filaments," by M. A. Bharier, et al. J BACTERIOL. 105:413-421, January, 1971.

"Electron microscopy of endoflagella and microtubules

in Treponema reiter," by K. H. Hougen, et al. ACTA PATHOL MICROBIOL SCAND. 79:37-50, 1971.

"Evaluation of the autoimmune response in syphilis by use of a modified Jerne method," by N. I. Tuma-sheva, et al. VESTN DERMATOL VENEROL. 45:62-64, November, 1971.

"Evaluation of the automated fluorescent treponema antibody test for syphilis," by H. J. Hornstein, et al. J LAB CLIN MED. 77:885-890, May, 1971.

"Evaluation of qualitative hemagglutination test for antibodies to Treponema pallidum," by R. A. Le Clair. J INFECT DIS. 123:668-670, June, 1971.

"Evaluation of the results of the leukocyte agglomer-ation test in syphilis," by IuA Rodin, et al. VESTN DERMATOL VENEROL. 45:64-68, November, 1971.

"FTA-ABS and VDRL slide test reactivity in a population of Nuns," by J. N. Goldman, et al. JAMA. 217:53-55, July 5, 1971.

"False positive Wassermann reaction associated with evidence of enterovirus infection," by R. A. Quaife, et al. J CLIN PATHOL. 24:120-121, March, 1971.

"Familial chronic biologic false-positive seroreactions for syphilis. Report of two families, one with three generations affected," by G. H. Kostant. JAMA. 219:45-48, January, 1972.

"Further evaluation of the automated fluorescent tre-ponemal antibody test for syphilis," by E. M. Coffey, et al. APPL MICROBIOL. 21:820-822, May, 1971.

"Immobilization effects of anticell and antiaxial fila-ment sera on Treponema zuelzerae," by M. A. Bharier, et al. J BACTERIOL. 105:430-437, January, 1971.

"Immunity conditions in treponematoses," by T. Guthe, et al. HAUTARZT. 22:329-333, August, 1971.

"Immunoelectrophoretic studies of immunoglobulins in early acquired syphilis," by M. Gibowski, et al. PRZEGL DERMATOL. 58:708-713, November - December, 1971.

"Immunofluorescence reaction using fresh blood in syphilis," by T. I. Milonova. VESTN DERMATOL VENER- OL. 45:68-73, February, 1971.

"Immunofluorescent staining for the detection of Tre- ponema pallidum in early syphilitic lesions," by A. E. Wilkinson, et al. BR J VENER DIS. 47:252- 254, August, 1971.

"Immunological patterns in syphilis including the question of antibodies," by H. Grossmann, et al. HAUTARZT. 21:245-252, June, 1970.

"Immunological studies on treponemal antigens. II. Serological changes and resistance to infection in rabbits immunized with culture supernatant of aviru- lent Treponema pallidum," by N. N. Izzat, et al. BR J VENER DIS. 47:335-338, October, 1971.

"Incomplete agglutinins against Treponema pallidum," by J. Podwinska, et al. BR J VENER DIS. 47:81-86, April, 1971.

"Keratodermia blenorrhagica in Reiter's disease," by R. Howell. BR MED J. 1:725-726, March 27, 1971.

"Lipid metabolism in the parasitic and free-living spirochetes Treponema pallidum (Reiter) and Tre- ponema zuelzerae," by H. Meyer, et al. BIOCHIM

BIOPHYS ACTA. 231:93-106, February 2, 1971.

"The luminescent method of detecting pupillary disorders in early forms of syphilis," by V. D.
Kochetkov, et al. ZH NEVROPATOL PSIKHIATR. 71:202-
204, 1971.

"Lymphoblastic transformation test during syphilis,"
by C. Janot, et al. PRESSE MED. 79:1901-1904,
October 16, 1971.

"Masking of syphilis." BR MED J. 3:206, July 24, 1971.

"Metronidazole as a possible reason for difficulty in
diagnosis of syphilis," by I. I. I'lin, et al. VESTN
DERMATOL VENEROL. 45:74-76, February, 1971.

"Microreaction on glass with fresh blood, plasma and
active serum in syphilis," by T. I. Milonova, et
al. VESTN DERMATOL VENEROL. 45:40-44, May, 1971.

"Occurrence of fetal syphilis after a nonreactive
early gestational serologic test," by F. L. al-Salihi
et al. J PEDIATR. 78:121-123, January, 1971.

"Occurrence of latent forms of syphilis in the absence
of manifestations in the beginning stages," by S.
I. Berlin, et al. VESTN DERMATOL VENEROL. 45:45-
50, May, 1971.

"1 of the causes of nonspecific false positive reaction
in syphilis," by L. G. Sagdeeva. VESTN DERMATOL
VENEROL. 44:59-64, September, 1970.

"Physiologic changes during the Jarisch-Herxheimer reaction in early syphilis. A comparison with louse-
borne relapsing fever," by D. A. Warrell, et al.
AM J MED. 51:176-185, August, 1971.

SYPHILIS: DIAGNOSIS

"Practical interpretation of serologic tests for
syphilis," by M. Renoux. PRESSE MED. 79:685-689,
March 24, 1971.

"A preliminary study of the treponemal pallidum haemagglutination test (TPHA)," by S. Vejjajiva, et al.
J MED ASSOC THAI. 54:256-259, April, 1971.

"Principle and effect of anti-treponema pallida specific
syphilis tests FTA and TPI," by G. Blaurock, et al.
DTSCH GESUNDHEITSW. 26:1152-1156, June 17, 1971.

"Problem of latent syphilis," by L. A. Rozina, et al.
VESTN DERMATOL VENEROL. 45:57-59, June, 1971.

"Proteinogram and results of immunofluorescence tests
in the examination of dried sera of patients with
syphilis," by S. M. Vorobeichik, et al. VESTN DER-
MATOL VENEROL. 45:45-50, October, 1971.

"Quantitative determination and serological activity
of 19S-and 7S-immunoglobulins in syphilis," by E.
Kuwert, et al. Z IMMUNITAETSFORSCH EXP KLIN IMMUNOL.
141:303-316, April, 1971.

"Rapid plasma diagnosis of syphilis," by G. Nicolau,
et al. ROM MED REV. 15:44-48, January - March, 1971.

"Rapid plasma reagin (RPR) card test. A screening
method for treponemal disease," by A. N. Walker.
BR J VENER DIS. 47:259-262, August, 1971.

"Sensitivity and specificity of automated serologic
tests for syphilis," by T. R. Cate, et al. AM J
CLIN PATHOL. 55:735-739, June, 1971.

"Serologic diagnosis of lues," by C. Garofoli. POLI-
CLINICO. 78:452-460, June 1, 1971.

"Serologic syphilis reactions in the Tangiers region," by M. Mailloux. MAROC MED. 51:172-173, March, 1971.

"Serologic tests for syphilis diagnosis in general practice," by I. Racz. ORV HETIL. 112:630-631, March, 1971.

"Seroresistant syphilis," by N. M. Ovchinnikov. VESTN DERMATOL VENEROL. 45:35-41, August, 1971.

"Significance of the Nelson reaction in the diagnosis of syphilitic organ involvement," by J. Kozakiewicz, et al. POL TYG LEK. 26:706-708, May 10, 1971.

"A simplified schema for the evaluation of reactive serologic tests for syphilis," by L. Nicholas. J CHRONIC DIS. 24:281-284, August, 1971.

"Some unusual manifestations of syphilis. Condylomata lata of the face. A retrospective diagnosis," by V. N. Sehgal, et al. BR J VENER DIS. 47:204-205, June, 1971.

"Spurious manifestations of cerebral tumor in the course of hysterica reaction in a child with syphilitic encephalopathy," by A. Bratkowa. POL TYG LEK. 26:217-218, July 8, 1971.

"Sulphydryl sensitivity of syphilitic antibodies and temperature dependence in complement fixation," by M. Surjan, et al. BR J VENER DIS. 47:87-90, April, 1971.

"Syphilis diagnosis in the age of antibiotics," by A. Luger. WIEN KLIN WOCHENSCHR. 83:241-245, April 9, 1971.

"Temporary positiveness of the F.A.T. test in primary

syphilis during the course of treatment," by G. F.
Strani, et al. G ITAL DERMATOL. 46:334-335, July,
1971.

"Testing for congenital syphilis in interstitial keratitis," by J. L. Smith. AM J OPHTHALMOL. 72:816-
820, October, 1971.

"Treponema pallidum immobilization test in properly
treated patients with syphilis," by T. V. Vasil'ev,
et al. VESTN DERMATOL VENEROL. 45:52-57, June,
1971.

"Ultrastructure of Treponema pallidum Nichols following
lysis by physical and chemical methods. I. Envel-
ope, wall, membrane and fibrils," by S. Jackson, et
al. ARCH MIKROBIOL. 76:308-324, 1971.

--II. Axial filaments," by S. Jackson, et al. ARCH
MIKROBIOL. 76:325-340, 1971.

"The VDRL slide test in 322 cases of darkfield positive
primary syphilis," by R. D. Wende, et al. SOUTH
MED J. 64:633-634, May, 1971.

"The value of autoantibodies to vascular lipids in
syphilis and non-syphilis," by O. J. Stone. INT J
DERMATOL. 10:31-34, January-March, 1971.

"Value of the Treponema pallidum immobilization test
in the detection of late and visceral syphilis in
general hospital patients," by N. M. Ovchinnikov,
et al. VESTN DERMATOL VENEROL. 45:53-57, September,
1971.

"Venereal disease. Acquired syphilis--drugs and blood
tests," by W. J. Brn. AM J NURS. 71:713-715, April,
1971.

SYPHILIS: DIAGNOSIS: CEREBROSPINAL FLUID

"Examination of cerebrospinal fluid," by V. Cagli.
POLICLINICO. 78:466-474, June 1, 1971.

"Fluorescent treponemal antibody tests on cerebrospinal
fluid," by M. F. Garner, et al. BR J VENER DIS.
47:356-358, October, 1971.

"Immunoglobuline in cerebrospinal fluid. Syphilis and
IgG," by H. J. Heitmann. DTSCH MED WOCHENSCHR. 96:
966-967, May 28, 1971.

"Quantitative study of immunoglobulins in the cerebrospinal fluid of neuroluetics," by G. Martina, et
al. G ITAL DERMATOL. 46:322-323, July, 1971.

"Validity of the VDRL test on cerebrospinal fluid contaminated by blood," by N. N. Izzat, et al. BR J
VENER DIS. 47:162-164, June, 1971.

SYPHILIS: EXPERIMENTAL
"Elimination of intercurrent death among rabbits ino-
culated with Treponema pallidum," by H. J. Jensen.
ACTA PATHOL MICROBIOL SCAND. 79:124-125, 1971.

"Evolution of syphilitic chancres with virulent Treponema pallidum in the rabbit," by N. N. Izzat, et
al. BR J VENER DIS. 47:67-72, April, 1971.

"Resistance and serological changes in rabbits immunized
with virulent Treponema pallidum sonicate," by N.
N. Izzat, et al. ACTA DERM VENEREOL. 51:157-160,
1971.

"Serum, lymph node and testicular concentrations of
penicillin in 31 healthy or syphilitic rabbits treate
with penicillin," by J. C. Pechere, et al. PATHOL
BIOL. 19:49-52, January, 1971.

"Single-dose treatment of gonorrhoea with penicillin

SYPHILIS: EXPERIMENTAL

or thiamphenicol and its effect on T. pallidum in experimental syphilis," by D. Petzold. BR J VENER DIS. 47:380, October, 1971.

"Studies on Treponema pallidum haemagglutination antibodies. I. TPHA antibodies in experimental syphilitic rabbits," by S. Okamoto, et al. BR J VENER DIS. 47:77-80, April, 1971.

SYPHILIS: GASTROINTESTINAL

"Syphilis lesions of the stomach treated surgically," by A. Kulicz, et al. POL PRZEGL CHIR. 43:641-643, 1971.

SYPHILIS: HEPATIC

"Differential diagnosis of virus hepatitis against hepatic syphilis," by O. Granicki, et al. POL TYG LEK. 26:276-278, February 22, 1971.

"Early syphilitic hepatitis. A possible case," by R. A. LeClair. BR J VENER DIS. 47:212, June, 1971.

"Liver disease associated with early syphilis," by A. L. Baker, et al. N ENGL J MED. 284:1422-1423, June 24, 1971.

"Liver disease associated with secondary syphilis," by R. V. Lee, et al. N ENGL J MED. 284:1423-1425, June 24, 1971.

"The liver in secondary (early) syphilis," by S. Sherlock. N ENGL J MED. 284:1437-1438, June 24, 1971.

"Study of 2 cases of congenital syphilitic hepatitis with biopsy," by G. Lepercq, et al. ANN MED INTERNE. 122:633-638, May, 1971.

SYPHILIS: HISTORY

"Syphilis and Neanderthal man," by D. J. Wright. NATURE

SYPHILIS: HISTORY

(London). 229:409, February 5, 1971.

"Syphilis in the Bible," by L. Goldman. ARCH DERMATOL.
103:535-536, May, 1971.

"Syphilis in the Hutten skeleton. Last doubts on the
true identity of the skeleton discovered in 1968 on
the Ufenau island in Lake Zurich could be dissipated
through research," by H. Jung. HAUTARZT. 22:509,
November, 1971.

"Syphilis--1957 to 1970," by J. Murphree. J MED ASSOC
STATE ALA. 40:479-480, January, 1971.

SYPHILIS: NASOPHARYNGEAL
"Tertiary syphilis of the nasal fossa and the pharynx,"
by E. G. Tutor. ACTA OTORINOLARYNGOL IBER AM. 22:
366-384, 1971.

SYPHILIS: NEONATAL
"Congenital syphilis in the newborn infant: clinical
and pathological observations in recent cases," by
E. H. Oppenheimer, et al. JOHNS HOPKINS MED J.
129:63-82, August, 1971.

"Effects of the increasing frequency of adult contagious
syphilis on those of newborn infants and infants in
the Lille and Douai areas since 1962," by F. Desmons.
PEDIATRIE. 26:429-432, June, 1971.

"Neonatal congenital syphilis. Diagnosis by the anti
IgM treponemal fluorescence test," by J. Kipnis, et
al. REV INST MED TROP SAO PAULO. 13:179-183, May-
June, 1971.

SYPHILIS: NEUROSYPHILIS
"Analysis of hospital admission rates of patients with
syphilis of the central nervous system in Poland before and after World War II," by A. Dowzenko, et al.

POL MED J. 10:539-546, 1971.

"Autoimmune processes in neuropsychic diseases," by S.
F. Semenov. VESTN AKAD MED NAUK SSSR. 26:78-81,
1971.

"Case of congenital neurosyphilis with a picture of
juvenile progressive paralysis," by W. Nyka. NEURO-
PATOL POL. 9:353-357, October-December, 1971.

"Clinical progression of ocular syphilis and neurosyphilis despite treatment with massive doses of
penicillin. Failure to demonstrate treponemes in
affected tissues," by C. N. Sowmini. BR J VENER DIS.
47:348-355, October, 1971.

"Electro-clinical correlations in neurosyphilis," by
C. Postelnicu, et al. ELECTROENCEPHALOGR CLIN
NEUROPHYSIOL. 30:361, April, 1971.

"F.T.A. test in neurosyphilis. Immunologic studies with
fluorescent antiglobulins fractionated in serum and
in cerebrospinal fluid," by S. Sartoris, et al. G
ITAL DERMATOL. 46:330-331, July, 1971.

"Pathogenesis of pupillary disorders in various forms
of syphilis of the nervous system," by V. D. Kochetkov,
et al. VESTN DERMATOL VENEROL. 44:53-58, March,
1970.

"Polyneuritis in the course of early latent syphilis,"
by K. Hulanicka, et al. NEUROL NEUROCHIR POL. 5:
121-124, 1971.

"Review of hospitalized cases of general paralysis of
the insane," by K. Dawson-Butterworth, et al. BR
J VENER DIS. 46:295-302, August, 1970.

"Treatment of neurosyphilis," by J. Tempski-Templehof,

et al. HAREFUAH. 80:196-198, February 15, 1971.

SYPHILIS: OCCURRENCE
"Analysis of early syphilis incidence in the rural
environment of the Bialystok province between 1965
and 1969," by H. Szarmach, et al. PRZEGL DERMATOL.
58:279-286, May-June, 1971.

"Anatomical evidence of pre-columbian syphilis in the
West Indian Islands," by N. G. Gejvall, et al. AM
J OCCUP THER. 25:138-157, October, 1971.

"Endemic syphilis, venereal syphilis, diseases of the
civilization," by J. Tisseuil. BULL SOC PATHOL EXOT.
64:296-300, May-June, 1971.

"The incidence of syphilis in the Banut: survey of 587
cases from Baragwanath hospital," by M. Dogliotti.
S AFR MED J. 45:8-10, January 2, 1971.

"Seriologic and parasitologic survey in aboriginal
populations of the Republic of Rwanda. I. Results
of the seriologic survey. Frequency of syphilis in
aboriginal populations of the Republic of Rwanda.
II. Results of the parasitologic survey: protist
and filariae," by R. Biemans, et al. BULL SOC PATHOL
EXOT. 64:277-291, May-June, 1971.

"Syphilis among employees of the health service establishments treated at the Department of Dermatology
of the Medical Academy in Cracow in 1960-1969," by
Bogdaszewska-Czabanowska, et al. PRZEGL DERMATOL.
58:435-440, 1971.

"Syphilis in the Bundeswehr. Statistical evaluation
of documentations from the past 10 years," by H.
Biehler. HAUTARZT. 22:206-213, May, 1971.

"World-wide epidemiological tendencies of syphilis and

SYPHILIS: OCCURRENCE

blenorrhagia," by T. Guthe. BOL OF SANIT PANAM.
70:6-25, January, 1971.

SYPHILIS: OPHTHALMIC
"Acute choroido-retinitis in secondary syphilis. Presence of spiral organisms in the aqueous humour,"
by P. A. Macfaul, et al. BR J VENER DIS. 47:159-
161, June, 1971.

"Clinical progression of ocular syphilis and neurosyphilis despite treatment with massive doses of
penicillin. Failure to demonstrate treponemes in
affected tissues," by C. N. Sowmini. BR J VENER DIS.
47:348-355, October, 1971.

"Syphilitic chorio-retinitis: report of an active case,"
by M. A. Mohamed. BULL OPHTHALMOL SOC EGYPT. 63:
217-221, 1970.

"Syphilitic scleritis. Clinical and angiographic aspects," by F. Deodati, et al. BULL SOC OPHTALMOL
FR. 71:63-65, January, 1971.

SYPHILIS: ORAL
"A case of sero-positive primary syphilis of the tonsil," by N. H. Vincenti. J LARYNGOL OTOL. 85:869-
870, August, 1971.

SYPHILIS: OSSEOUS
"Early congenital bone syphilis: various clinical and
radiological aspects," by A. Fazzi, et al. REV PAUL
MED. 77:73-76, March, 1971.

SYPHILIS: PREGNANCY
"Changes in the trends in syphilis in pregancy," by C.
Sawazaki, et al. SANFUJINKA JISSAI. 20:112-119,
February, 1971.

"Fetal growth with congenital syphilis: a quantitative

study," by R. L. Naeye. AM J CLIN PATHOL. 55:228-231, February, 1971.

"Late results of a complex study of children born to syphilitic mothers properly treated before and during pregnancy," by P. E. Pochkhua. VESTN DERMATOL VENEROL. 45:66-67, February, 1971.

"Occurrence of fetal syphilis after a nonreactive early gestational seriologic test," by F. L. al-Salihi, et al. J PEDIATR. 78:121-123, January, 1971.

"Therapy for syphilis during pregnancy," by R. P. George, Jr. N ENGL J MED. 284:1271-1272, June 3, 1971.

SYPHILIS: PREVENTION AND CONTROL
"Eradication of syphilis," by S. Jonas, et al. N ENGL J MED. 285:412, August 12, 1971.

"The essential elements of a syphilis control program," by W. J. Brown. BOL OF SANIT PANAM. 70:59-65, January, 1971.

"Possibility of the transmission of syphilis in the blood of a donor with a latent form of this disease," by A. A. Mikhailova, et al. PROBL GEMATOL PERELIV KROVI. 16:50-51, July, 1971.

"Treatment and prevention of syphilis and gonorrhea." MED LETT DRUGS THER. 13:85-87, October, 1971.

SYPHILIS: PULMONARY
"Case of syphilis of the lung," by K. B. Ruszel. POL TYG LEK. 26:645-646, April 26, 1971.

"Syphilitic pulmonary infarct revealing gumma," by J. Vidal, et al. PRESSE MED. 79:763, April 3, 1971.

SYPHILIS: RENAL

"Nephropathy of secondary syphilis. A clinical and
pathological spectrum," by M. S. Bhorade, et al.
JAMA. 216:1159-1166, May 17, 1971.

SYPHILIS: SEROLOGY AND SERODIAGNOSIS
"Blood platelet behaviour in syphilis," by S. F.
Szanto. BR J VENER DIS. 47:14-16, February, 1971.

"Changes in the serum transaminases in patients with
syphilis," by B. S. Tio, et al. BR J VENER DIS.
47:263-265, August, 1971.

"Cortuitous discovery of a positive syphilitic serology
(attempted interpretation and management)," by M.
J. Maleville. BORD MED. 4:747-748, March, 1971.

"Detection of incomplete antibodies in the blood serum
of patients with infectious forms of syphilis and
some dermatoses," by L. S. Reznikova, et al. VESTN
DERMATOL VENEROL. 45:44-51, August, 1971.

"Diagnostic value of the Roemer and Schlïpkoeter test
in serodiagnosis of late syphilis," by L. Abate, et
al. ARCISP S ANNA FERRARA. 23:309-315, 1970.

"Evaluation of 'atypical' variants of the results in
the specific syphilis serology," by L. Krell, et al.
DTSCH GESUNDHEITSW. 26:1712-1716, September 2, 1971.

"Modern serology of syphilis. I. Preparation and testing of the cardiolipin antigen for the complement
fixation reaction, introduced in production at the
'Dr. I. Cantacuzino Institute'," by M. Georgescu,
et al. MICROBIOL PARAZITOL EPIDEMIOL. 16:67-72,
January-February, 1971.

--II. Preparation for production of a cardiolipin
antigen of the VDRL type for serodiagnosis of
syphilis with a flocculation reaction. Value and

methods of use," by M. Georgescu, et al. MICROBIOL
PARAZITOL EPIDEMIOL. 16:263-272, May-June, 1971.

"Serology of syphilis. Development and concepts.
Study on 50 patients," by L. Belli, et al. PRENSA
MED ARGENT. 58:720-725, June 4, 1971.

"Syphilis reference serology," by A. Fischman, et al.
NZ MED J. 74:238-240, October, 1971.

"Syphilis serodiagnosis, with special reference to
FTA-ABS and TPHA," by H. Ota, et al. J JAP ASSOC
INFECT DIS. 45:112-115, March, 1971.

"Value of present-day serological tests in the diagnosis
of symptomless sources of infection and contacts in
early syphilis," by W. Manikowska-Lesinska, et al.
PRZEGL DERMATOL. 58:157-162, March-April, 1971.

SYPHILIS: TREATMENT
"Adequate treatment for syphilis," by G. Allyn. ARCH
DERMATOL. 103:462, April, 1971.

"Blood level studies on the depot effect of clemizole-
penicillin G in antiluetic therapy," by D. Kleinhans.
Z HAUT GESCHLECHTSKR. 46:359-365, June 1, 1971.

"A case of failure in the treatment of early syphilis
with erythromycin," by Z. Dratwinski. PRZEGL DER-
MATOL. 58:69-71, January-February, 1971.

"Clinico-prognostic significance of the Treponema
pallidum immobilization reaction in patients with
seroresistant syphilis," by IuK Skripkin, et al.
VESTN DERMATOL VENEROL. 45:58-62, January, 1971.

"Continuous penicillin therapy of patients with infectious syphilis," by M. P. Frishman, et al. VESTN
DERMATOL VENEROL. 44:52-57, September, 1970.

"Continuous treatment of early forms of syphilis with penicillin and bicillin," by Iuf Korolev. VOEN MED ZH. 7:76-77, 1971.

"Current features in current syphilis therapy," by V. A. Rudaev. FELDSHER AKUSH. 36:26-29, August, 1971.

"Dynamics of antibody subsidence in early symptomatic syphilis treated with penicillin," by I. Kiersnicka-Itman, et al. PRZEGL DERMATOL. 58:699-707, November-December, 1971.

"Effect of penicillin and bicillin-1 in experimental syphilis in rabbits," by N. M. Ovchinnikov, et al. VESTN DERMATOL VENEROL. 45:42-47, June, 1971.

"Hyaluronidase activity as a factor of vascular permeability in patients with syphilis during treatment," by V. V. Kalugin, et al. VESTN DERMATOL VENEROL. 45:56-60, October, 1971.

"Immediate results of bicillin-5 treatment of patients with infectious forms of syphilis," by S. H. Khamidov. VESTN DERMATOL VENEROL. 45:41-44, August, 1971.

"Late results of treating syphilis with bicillin-1,3,4 and bicillin-3,4 in combination with pyrogenal," by T. V. Vasil'ev. VESTN DERMATOL VENEROL. 45:50-58, January, 1971.

"The Nelson-Mayer TPI-test and the treatment of syphilis in medical practice," by K. Hubschmann. WIEN KLIN WOCHENSCHR. 82:371-373, May 15, 1970.

"Ominous follow-up to syphilis." MED WORLD NEWS. 12:16-17, January 29, 1971.

"Pathogenesis and treatment of seroresistant syphilis," by A. A. Studnitsin, et al. VESTN DERMATOL VENEROL.

45:47-52, June, 1971.

"Penicillin therapy in 44 cases of primary and secondary syphilis," by B. A. Smithurst. MED J AUST. 2:
248-250, July 31, 1971.

"Persistence of T. pallidum and its significance in
penicillin-treated seropositive late syphilis," by
L. Yogeswari, et al. BR J VENER DIS. 47:339-349,
October, 1971.

"Reappearance of soft chancre (5 cases)," by H. Perrot,
et al. BULL SOC FR DERMATOL SYPHILIGR. 78:200-201,
1971; also in: LYON MED. 225:649-650, April 11,
1971.

"Re-appraising the effect on incubating syphilis of
treatment for gonorrhoea," by K. R. Woodcock. BR
J VENER DIS. 47:95-101, April, 1971.

"Recurrence of soft chancre. 2 recent cases," by D.
Colomb, et al. BULL SOC FR DERMATOL SYPHILIGR. 78:
197-199, 1971.

"Repeated syphilis infection after treatment by a permanent method," by M. Z. Kagan, et al. VESTN DERMA-
TOL VENEROL. 45:76-79, September, 1971.

"Results of electroencephalography in early and latent
syphilis," by N. V. Bratus', et al. VESTN DERMATOL
VENEROL. 45:50-53, July, 1971.

"Site of action of efficacy of anti-syphilitic treatment
with penicillin. II. Problems of penicillin dosage,"
by A. Luger. HAUTARZT. 22:1-6, January, 1971.

"Therapy for incubating syphilis. Effectiveness of
gonorrhea treatment," by A. L. Schroeter, et al.
JAMA. 218:711-713, November 1, 1971.

SYPHILIS: TREATMENT

"Therapy for syphilis during pregnancy," by R. P.
George, Jr. N ENGL J MED. 284:1271-1272, June 3,
1971.

"Therapy of syphilis at the Prague Medical Clinic in
the year 1824," by L. Sinkulova. CESK DERMATOL.
46:87-90, April, 1971.

"3 cases of resistance to antisyphilitic treatment,"
by KhN Khidyrov, et al. VESTN DERMATOL VENEROL.
44:57-59, September, 1970.

"Treatment of early syphilis and venereal lymphogranu-
lomatosis with doxycycline," by H. Hevia, et al.
REV MED CHIL. 99:402-405, June, 1971.

"Unsuccessful treatment of early symptomatic syphilis
following oral administration of detreomycin, erythromycin and oxyterracin," by J. Lebioda, et al.
PRZEGL LEK. 27:469-472, 1971.

"An unusual Jarisch-Herxheimer reaction," by R. N. Thin.
BR J VENER DIS. 47:293-294, August, 1971.

TABES
"Abnormal chemoreceptor response to hypoxia in patients
with tabes dorsalis," by R. J. Evans, et al. BR
MED J. 1:530-531, March 6, 1971.

"Case of progressive course of tabes dorsalis despite
penicillin treatment and disappearance of changes
in cerebrospinal fluid," by H. Wisniewski, et al.
NEUROL NEUROCHIR POL. 5:237-239, 1971.

TESTS AND DIAGNOSIS
"Apparent transient false-positive FTA-ABS test following smallpox vaccination." J OKLA STATE MED ASSOC.
64:372, September, 1971.

"Atypical FTA-ABS test fluorescence in lupus erythematosus," by F. Jennis. JAMA. 215:588-589, January 18, 1971.

"Atypical FTA-ABS test reaction. An initial clue in the diagnosis of lupus erythematosus," by S. J. Kraus, et al. ARCH DERMATOL. 104:260-261, September, 1971.

"Atypical fluorescence in the fluorescent treponemal-antibody-absorption (FTA-ABS) test related to deoxyribonucleic acid (DNA) antibodies," by S. J. Kraus, et al. J IMMUNOL. 106:1665-1669, June, 1971

"Automation of the Wassermann complement-fixation test using a discrete analyser," by J. H. Glenn, et al. BR J VENER DIS. 47:200-203, June, 1971.

"CBC done--no VDRL results: two congenital syphilitics," by H. P. Hines, et al. JAP J PHYSIOL. 67:309-310, July, 1971.

"Characteristics of fluorescein labelled antiglobulin preparations that may affect the fluorescent treponemal antibody-absorption test," by P. H. Hardy, et al. AM J CLIN PATHOL. 56:181-186, August, 1971.

"Clinical evaluation of the T. pallidum haemagglutinati test," by T. Uete, et al. BR J VENER DIS. 47:73-76, April, 1971.

"Current epidemiological value of prophylactic serological tests," by J. Lesinski, et al. PRZEGL DERMA TOL. 58:163-168, March-April, 1971.

"A laboratory test is not a diagnosis," by N. J. Fiumara JAMA. 217:71, July 5, 1971.

"A lyophilization medium for FTA-ABS test antigen," by

E. F. Hunter, et al. HEALTH LAB SCI. 8:35-39, January, 1971.

"A lyophilization medium for FTA-ABS test antigen," by E. F. Hunter, et al. HEALTH LAB SCI. 8:35-39, January, 1971.

"'Microtiter' technic for VDRL," by S. S. Kasatiya, et al. CAN J PUBLIC HEALTH. 62:61-62, January-February, 1971.

"Positive fluorescent treponemal antibody test in systemic lupus erythematosus in childhood: report of a case," by R. P. Lesser, et al. J PEDIATR. 79: 1006-1008, December, 1971.

"Practical evaluation of culture media with SCA basis produced by the Serology and Vaccine Institute," by V. Resl, Jr. CESK DERMATOL. 46:29-38, February, 1971.

"Practical interpretation of serologic tests for syphilis," by M. Renoux. PRESSE MED. 79:685-689, March 24, 1971.

"A preliminary study of the treponemal pallidum haemagglutination test (TPHA)," by S. Vejjajiva, et al. J MED ASSOC THAI. 54:256-259, April, 1971.

"Results of the Nelson test during administration of gentamycin," by H. J. Heitmann, et al. Z HAUT GESCHLECHTSKR. 46:87-90, February 1, 1971.

"The role of sorbent in the absorbed fluorescent treponemal antibody (FTA-ABS) test," by A. E. Wilkinson, et al. PROC R SOC MED. 64:422-425, April, 1971.

"The significance of cardiolipin immunofluorescence," by J. M. Wright, et al. PROC R SOC MED. 64:419-422,

TESTS AND DIAGNOSIS

April, 1971.

"Significance of the lymphocyte transformation test in dermatology," by N. Simon, et al. BERUFSDERMATOSEN. 18:189-219, August, 1970.

"Specificity of the FTA-200 test and the FTA-ABS test," by B. Evelk. HAUTARZT. 22:442-445, October, 1971.

TETRACYCLINE

"Balanitis due to fixed drug eruption associated with tetracycline therapy," by G. W. Csonka, et al. BR J VENER DIS. 47:42-44, February, 1971.

"The effect of antibiotic therapy on mycoplasma in the female genital tract. In vitro and in vivo studies on the sensitivity of Mycoplasma hominis and T-mycoplasmas to tetracyclines and other antibiotics," by L. Westrom, et al. ACTA OBSTET GYNECOL SCAND. 50:25-31, 1971.

"Tetracycline in pregnancy?" by B. G. Newman. ANN INTERN MED. 75:648-649, October, 1971.

"Tetracycline inhibition of Mycoplasma ribosomal protein synthesis," by C. C. Fraterrigo, et al. J ANTIBIOT. 24:185-188, March, 1971.

"Therapy of gonorrhea with tetracycline," by J. Danda. CESK DERMATOL. 46:1-6, February, 1971.

"Treatment of gonorrhoea with two oral doses of antibiotics. Trials of cephalexin and of triple tetracycline," by R. R. Willcox. BR J VENER DIS. 47:31-33, February, 1971.

"Treatment of gynecologic infections by combined tetracycline and amphotericin B," by M. Van Gijsegem. BRUX MED. 51:391-393, May, 1971.

THIAMPHENICOL

"Single-dose treatment of gonorrhoea with penicillin
or thiamphenicol and its effect on T. pallidum in
experimental syphilis," by D. Petzold. BR J VENER
DIS. 47:380, October, 1971.

"Use of single doses of thiamphenicol in gonoccocal
urethritis," by V. Rodrigues, et al. REV BRAS MED.
28:288-290, June, 1971.

THRUSH COLPITIS
See: Colpitis

TINIDAZOLE
"Treatment of trichomonas infections with tinidazol in
women," by J. Diwald. WIEN MED WOCHENSCHR. 121:
492-494, June 12, 1971.

TORULOPSIS
"Relationship of Torulopsis to candida," by B. G. Leask,
et al. LANCET. 1:1300-1301, June 19, 1971.

TREATMENT
"Management of sexually assaulted females," by J. B.
Massey, et al. OBSTET GYNECOL. 38:29-36, July,
1971.

"Prophylactic treatment with penicillin in venereal
diseases," by A. Luger. HAUTARZT. 22:135, March,
1971.

"Sexual behaviour of male Pakistanis attending venereal
disease clinics in Great Britain," by A. S. Hossain.
SOC SCI MED. 5:227-241, June, 1971.

"Single dose cures 96% of VD cases." AM DRUGGIST. 163:
62-63, June 14, 1971.

"Therapeutic tips in dermatological practice," by R.

TREATMENT

Schuppli. DERMATOLOGICA. 142:286-289, 1971.

"Therapy of venereal infections," by H. J. Heite. Z
ALLGEMEINMED. 47:457-462, March 31, 1971.

"Treatment of venereal diseases," by M. Janner. Z
ALLGEMEINMED. 47:891-899, June 20, 1971.

TRICHOMONIASIS
"About a new medium for culture of Trichomonas vaginalis," by N. Jankov, et al. FOLIA MED. 13:137-
140, 1971.

"Chemotherapeutic activity of liutenurin in experimental
trichomoniasis of white mice," by M. A. Rubinchik,
et al. MED PARAZITOL. 40:197-201, March-April,
1971.

"Clinical picture of combined gonorrheal-trichomonad
urethritis," by I. I. Mavrov, et al. VESTN DERMATOL
VENEROL. 45:84-86, June, 1971.

"Comparative microscopy, culture and serology studies
on Trichomonas vaginalis," by K. J. Beck, et al.
GEBURTSHILFE FRAUENHEIKD. 31:551-560, June, 1971.

"Complement-fixing antibodies to Bedsonia in Reiter's
syndrome, TRIC agent infection, and control groups,"
by J. Schachter. AM J OPHTHALMOL. 71:857-860,
April, 1971.

"Current problems concerning trichomoniasis," by R.
Bredland. TIDSSKR NOR LAEGEFOREN. 91:379-381,
February 20, 1971.

"Demonstration of the allergic delayed-reaction type
in mice following sensitization with Trichomonas
vaginalis and a further contribution on the specif-
city of the peritoneal cell reaction," by R. Michel.

Z TROPENMED PARASITOL. 22:91-97, March, 1971.

"Demonstration of the endocytosis process and lysosome structures in Trichomonas vaginalis," by G. Brugerolle. C R ACAD SCI. 272:2558-2560, May 17, 1971.

"Detection of the antitrichomonal drug nitrimidazine (Naxogin) in urine," by G. D. Morrison, et al. BR J VENER DIS. 47:38-39, February, 1971.

"Detection of Trichomonas vaginalis in patients with complaints of leukorrhea and the effects of treatment with methylmercadone at the Kurume University," by S. Kato, et al. SANFUJINKA JISSAI. 20:884-889, August, 1971.

"Effect of different immunization procedures on agglutination and precipitation reactions of Trichomonas galliae," by B. M. Honigberg, et al. J PARASITOL. 57:363-369, April, 1971.

"In vivo resistance to metronidazole induced on four recently isolated strains of Trichomonas vaginalis," by I. De Carneri, et al. ARZNEIM FORSCH. 21:377-381, March, 1971.

"The incidence of trichomoniasis and dysuria in pregnant women in eastern Uganda," by S. L. Lightman, et al. TROP GEOGR MED. 23:113-114, March, 1971.

"The maltose metabolism of Trichomonas gallinae (Rivolta, 1878). II. Metabolic studies," by J. J. Daly. J PARASITOL. 57:370-374, April, 1971.

"Nitrimidazine in the treatment of trichomonas vaginalis vaginitis," by L. Cohen. BR J VENER DIS. 47:177-178, June, 1971.

"Nitrimidazine in the treatment of trichomoniasis," by

TRICHOMONIASIS

M. Moffett, et al. BR J VENER DIS. 47:173-176, June, 1971.

"On the ultrastructure of Trichomonas vaginalis," by D. Panaitescu, et al. ARCH ROUM PATHOL EXP MICRO-BIOL. 30:87-106, March, 1971.

"Possibilities in influencing the occurrence of tricho-moniasis," by M. Valent. BRATISL LEK LISTY. 56: 21-28, 1971.

"Some enzyme and isoenzyme activities in Trichomonas vaginalis," by M. Chyle, et al. FOLIA MICROBIOL. 16:142-143, 1971.

"Some enzymes and isoenzymes of Trichomonas vaginalis and changes in their activities after inoculation with live mamalian virus," by M. Chyle, et al. CAS LEK CESK. 110:234-236, March, 1971.

"Squibb's amphotericin B in treatment of Candida albi-cans and Trichomonas vaginalis infections," by D. Panaitescu, et al. ARCH ROUM PATHOL EXP MICROBIOL. 30:79-86, March, 1971.

"Sterility in urogenital trichomoniasis," by J. Schmor. WIEN MED WOCHENSCHR. 120:808-812, November 14, 1971

"Strains of Trichomonas vaginalis resistant to metro-nidazole," by L. M. Korik. VESTN DERMATOL VENEROL. 45:77-80, January, 1971.

"Trichomoniasis of the paranasal sinuses," by E. Teisar et al. OTORINOLARINGOLOGIE. 16:265-269, July - Aug ust, 1971.

TRICHOMONIASIS: CHILDREN AND INFANTS
"Occurrence of Trichomonas vaginalis in the urinary system of newborn male infants," by Z. Worwag. WIAD

TRICHOMONIASIS: CHILDREN AND INFANTS

    PARAZYTOL. 17:351-354, 1971.

TRICHOMONIASIS: DIAGNOSIS
"Investigations on cultivation and biology of Tricho-
    monas vaginalis," by P. Christoe. ZENTRALBL BAK-
    TERIOL. 217:540-553, August, 1971.

"Morphologic and histochemical changes in the mucosa
    of the urogenital tract in gonorrhea, trichomonas
    and candidiasis," by V. G. Bilik, et al. VESTN
    DERMATOL VENEROL. 45:50-53, May, 1971.

"New method of staining Trichomonas," by P. Francec-
    hini. PRESSE MED. 79:486-487, February 27, 1971.

TRICHOMONIASIS: EXPERIMENTAL
"The isolation of trichomonads from pigeons," by T. M.
    Grimes, et al. AUST VET J. 47:160-161, April, 1971.

TRICHOMONIASIS: OCCURRENCE
"Incidence of Trichomonas vaginalis and of aspecific
    vaginitis in an apparently healthy female population.
    Colposcopic and cytological aspects," by B. Cuscianna,
    et al. MINERVA GINECOL. 23:270-272, March 31, 1971.

"Incidence of Trichomonas vaginalis infection in the
    female population of Santiago," by H. Schenone, et
    al. BOL CHIL PARASITOL. 24:159, July-December,
    1969.

"Incidence of vaginal trichomoniasis and microbial
    flora in hysterectomized patients," by J. M. Arizaga
    Cruz, et al. GINECOL OBSTET MEX. 29:271-274,
    March, 1971.

TRICHOMONIASIS: PREGNANCY
"The incidence of trichomoniasis and dysuria in pregnant
    women in Eastern Uganda," by S. L. Lightman, et al.
    TROP GEOGR MED. 23:113-114, March, 1971.

TRICHOMONIASIS: PREGNANCY

"Infection of the urinary system with Trichomonas
vaginalis in newborn female infants," by Z. Worwag.
WIAD PARAZYTOL. 17:355-358, 1971.

TRICHOMONIASIS: TREATMENT
"Evaluation of a new oral trichomonicid," by J. Delgado
Urdapilleta, et al. GINECOL OBSTET MEX. 29:515-
519, May, 1971.

"Experiments on the influence of metabolites and anti-
metabolites on the model of Trichomonas vaginalis.
I. Experiments with the vitamin-B 2-complex," by
C. P. Christow. ZENTRALBL BAKTERIOL. 217:381-402,
July, 1971.

"Life cycle of urogenital trichomonas under the influence of some chemicals," by I. K. Padchenko. PEDIAT
AKUSH GINEKOL. 2:53-55, 1971.

"Study of the trichomonacidal properties of pyrithione
(1-hydroxy-2-(1,H)-pyridinethione sodium salt)," by
R. Cavier, et al. ANN PHARM FR. 29:211-214, March,
1971.

"Treatment of trichomonas infections with tinidazol
in women," by J. Diwald. WIEN MED WOCHENSCHR. 121:
492-494, June 12, 1971.

"Treatment of trichomoniasis in the female with a 5-day
course of metronidazole (Flagyl)," by A. N. McClean.
BR J VENER DIS. 47:36-37, February, 1971.

"Treatment of trichomoniasis vaginalis," by H. Heiss.
WIEN MED WOCHENSCHR. 121:30-33, January 16, 1971.

"Treatment of vaginal trichomoniasis with takimetol
tablets (metronidazole preparation)," by H. Ishikawa
et al. SANFUJINKA JISSAI. 20:99-103, January, 1971

TRICHOMONIASIS: TREATMENT

"Trichomonas and oxytetracycline," by S. Szanto. BR
MED J. 2:467, May 22, 1971.

"Trichomoniasis in a closed community: Efficacy of
metronidazole," by E. E. Keighley. BR MED J. 1:
207-209, January 23, 1971.

TRICHOMYCIN
"Pyrolysis-gas chromatography of polyene antifungal
antibiotics: The nature of candicidin, levorin and
trichomycin," by H. J. Burrows, et al. J CHROMATOGR.
53:566-571, December 23, 1971.

TRIMETHOPRIM-SULFAMETHOXAZOLE
"Gonorrhea in women: treatment with sulfamethoxazole
and trimethoprim," by C. B. Schofield, et al. J
INFECT DIS. 124:533-538, December, 1971.

"Results of treatment with trimethoprim-sulfamethoxazole
in dermovenereology," by S. D. Randazzo. G ITAL
DERMATOL. 46:269-272, June, 1971.

"Trimethoprim-sulphamethoxazole in gonorrhoea," by S.
Ullman, et al. ACTA DERM VENEROL. 51:394-396, 1971.

"Trimethoprim-sulphamethoxazole (Septrin) in the treatment of rectal gonorrhoea," by M. A. Waugh. BR J
VENER DIS. 47:34-35, February, 1971.

"Uncomplicated gonorrhea treated with Trimethoprim and
sulphamethoxazole," by B. L. Jorgensen, et al. UGESKR
LAEGER. 133:1259-1260, July 2, 1971.

URETHRITIS: NON-SPECIFIC AND NON-GONORRHEAL
"Diagnosis and therapy of male urethritis," by J. Meyer-
Rohn. Z HAUT GESCHLECHTSKR. 46:153-158, March 1,
1971.

"Doxycycline treatment of nongonococcal urethritis with

special reference to T-strain mycoplasmas," by A. Lassus, et al. BR J VENER DIS. 47:126-130, April, 1971.

"Efficacy of prolonged regimes of oxytetracycline in the treatment of nongonococcal urethritis," by J. John. BR J VENER DIS. 47:266-268, August, 1971.

"Frenulumplasty: a method for prophylactic treatment in women with recurring urethritis after coitus," by A. Ingelman-Sundberg. NORD MED. 86:988-989, August 19, 1971.

"Genital herpes infection and non-specific urethritis," by S. Jeansson, et al. BR MED J. 3:247, July 24, 1971.

"Haemagglutination by the TRIC group of Chlamydia," by P. F. Elvin-Lewis, et al. J MED MICROBIOL. 4:31-41, February, 1971.

"Isolation of human genital TRIC agents in nongonococcal urethritis and Reiter's disease by an irradiated cell culture method," by D. K. Ford, et al. BR J VENER DIS. 47:196-197, June, 1971.

"Local treatment of female urethritis," by S. Nilsson. LAKARTIDNINGEN. 68:581-584, February 3, 1971.

"Management of nonspecific urethritis." BR MED J. 3:62, July 10, 1971.

"A note on congenital abnormalities of the penis. Incidence and relationship to urethritis," by A. I. Morrison. BR J VENER DIS. 47:182-183, June, 1971.

"Studies on T-strain mycoplasmas in nongonococcal urethritis," by E. Jansson, et al. BR J VENER DIS. 47:122-125, April, 1971.

URETHRITIS: NON-SPECIFIC AND NON-GONORRHEAL

"Study of mycoplasma in university students with non-gonococcal urethritis," by S. Sueltmann, et al. HEALTH LAB SCI. 8:62-66, April, 1971.

"T-strains of mycoplasma and nongonococcal urethritis," by H. Haas, et al. BR J VENER DIS. 47:131-134, April, 1971.

"Urethritis in male children," by D. I. Williams, et al. PROC R SOC MED. 64:133-134, February, 1971.

URTICARIA
"An assessment of the role of Candida albicans and food yeasts in chronic urticaria," by J. James, et al. BR J DERMATOL. 84:227-237, March, 1971.

VACCINATIONS AND VD
"Apparent transient false-positive FTA-ABS test following smallpox vaccination." J OKLA STATE MED ASSOC. 64:372, September, 1971.

VAGINITIS
"Administration of oxytetracycline hydrochloride with hydrocortisone (Oxycort Aerosol) in the treatment of non-specific vaginitis," by A. Ostrzenski. POL TYG LEK. 26:283-284, February 22, 1971.

"Arthritis, vaginitis and cardiac murmur," by S. Jacobs. J LA STATE MED SOC. 123:179-182, May, 1971.

"Chronic monilial vaginitis," by H. Hosen. ANN ALLERGY. 29:499, September, 1971.

"Clinical pharmacological aspects of a new hormone derivative (3-tetrahydropyranyl ether of 17-beta-estradiol)," by C. Andreoli, et al. MINERVA GINECOL. 23:711-724, September 30, 1971.

"Corynebacterium vaginale vaginitis in pregnant women,"

by J. F. Lewis, et al. AM J CLIN PATHOL. 56:580-583, November, 1971.

"Meningococci in vaginitis," by J. E. Gregory, et al. AM J DIS CHILD. 121:423, May, 1971.

"Meningococcus and gonococcus: never the Twain--well, hardly ever," by H. A. Feldman. N ENGL J MED. 285: 518-520, August 26, 1971.

"A new treatment for monilial vaginitis." PRACTITIONER. 207:236-238, August, 1971.

"Postirradiation vaginitis. An evaluation of prophylaxi with topical estrogen," by R. M. Pitkin, et al. RADIOLOGY. 99:417-421, May, 1971.

"Simultaneous infection of urinary tract and external genital organs in young and adolescent girls," by K. Vesely. GYNECOL PRAT. 22:191-192, 1971.

"Thoughts on the treatment of vaginitis," by G. W. Gray. J MED ASSOC STATE ALA. 41:79, August, 1971.

"Treatment of vaginitis of diverse etiology with pi-maricin," by F. Bianchi. MINERVA GINECOL. 23: 489-492, May 31, 1971.

"Treatment of vaginal fluor," by G. Kummel. MED WELT. 2:65-66, January 9, 1971.

"Treatment possibilities in fluor genitalis in derma-tological practice," by H. Weitgasser. Z HAUT GESCHLECHTSKR. 46:107-110, February 15, 1971.

"2 cases of vaginitis due to an as yet unknown parasite in gynecologic pathology," by M. Gaudefroy, et al. J SCI MED LILLE. 89:301-302, August-September, 1971.

VAGINITIS

"Vaginitis and tights," by J. Stallworthy. BR MED J.
2:108, April 10, 1971.

VENEREAL DISEASE
"Advances in the study of venereal disease," by A. J.
King. BR J CLIN PRACT. 25:295-301, July, 1971.

"Advances in the treatment of sexually transmitted
diseases," by R. D. Catterall. PRACTITIONER. 207:
516-523, October, 1971.

"Bacterial hitch-hikers," by T. L. Howard. J UROL.
106:94, July, 1971.

"Basic results of scientific research on the problem
of scientific bases of dermatology and venereology
for 1969," by N. M. Turanov, et al. VESTN DERMATOL
VENEROL. 44:7-13, September, 1970.

"The clock is ticking," by M. Strage. TODAY'S HEALTH.
49:16-18 plus, April, 1971.

"Dangers of venereal disease in the family," by S.
Chiritescu. MUNCA SANIT. 19:477-484, August, 1971.

"Epidemic spread." WORLD HEALTH. May, 1971, p. 13.

"Haemophilus influenzae infections of the genital tract,"
by R. J. Farrand. J MED MICROBIOL. 4:357-358,
August, 1971.

"Growing menace of VD," by M. Walker. TIMES EDUC SUP.
2948:36, November 19, 1971.

"The health of women," by J. Peel. BR MED J. 3:267-
271, July 31, 1971.

"The high price to pay for permissiveness," by B.
Keenan. OBSERVER. August 8, 1971, p. 20.

VENEREAL DISEASE

"The increase in venereal disease," by L. Cohn. MED J AUST. 1:171-172, January 16, 1971.

"Meet the VD epidemiologist," by D. C. Vandermeer. AM J NURS. 71:722-723, April, 1971.

"Mpilo Hospital Round. Euthyroidism, exophthalmos, acropachy and pretibial myxoedema," by J. E. Thomas. CENT AFR J MED. 17:23-24, January, 1971.

"Other sexually transmitted diseases. I.," by C. S. Nicol. BR MED J. 2:448-449, May 22, 1971.

--II. by C. S. Nicol. BR MED J. 2:507-509, May, 1971.

"Polyester sponge swabs to facilitate examination for genital infection in women," by J. K. Oates, et al. BR J VENER DIS. 47:289-292, August, 1971.

"The problem of venereal diseases in the Americas," by A. Llopis. BOL OF SANIT PANAM. 70:26-58, January, 1971.

"The problem of venereal diseases in Singapore," by R. S. Morton. BR J VENER DIS. 47:48-51, February, 1971.

"Problems in social medicine," by V. H. Wallace. MED J AUST. 2:828-829, October 16, 1971.

"Pruritus vulvae," by C. N. Hudson. BR MED J. 1: 656-657, March 20, 1971.

"The sexually transmitted diseases," by C. S. Nicol. PRACTITIONER. 206:277-279, February, 1971.

"Sexually transmitted infections," by V. T. Searle-Jordan. HUMANIST. 86:262-264, September, 1971.

"Sexually transmitted infections in the schoolchild,"
by J. L. Fluker. MIDWIFE HEALTH VISIT. 6:91-96,
March, 1970.

"She may look clean, but...." EMERGENCY MED. 3:98-
101 plus, March, 1971.

"The silent epidemic--venereal disease," by H. Pariser.
VA MED MON. 98:635-636, December, 1971.

"Specimens from the female genital tract," by S. Selwyn,
et al. BR MED J. 4:559-560, November 27, 1971.

"Statement on venereal disease." J KANS MED SOC. 72:
332, July, 1971.

"The unmentionable diseases," by K. Dicker. NURS TIMES.
67:94 plus, January 21, 1971.

"VD," by A. Blanzaco. TODAY'S EDUC. 60:41, December,
1971.

"VD," by H. Miller. LISTENER. 86:572, October 28,
1971.

"VD: the clock is ticking," by M. Strage. TODAY'S
HEALTH. 49:16-18 plus, April, 1971.

"VD: a national epidemic." MED TIMES. 99:109, May,
1971.

"VD statistics," by A. S. Wigfield. BR MED J. 4:
750, December 18, 1971.

"Venereal disease." SOUTH MED J. 64:1157-1158,
September, 1971.

"Venereal disease," by F. W. Barton. JAMA. 216:1472-

1473, May 31, 1971.

"Venereal disease," by T. H. Bierre. OCCUP HEALTH. 4:3-4, December, 1970.

"Venereal disease," by D. Rubin. MCCALLS. 98:64 plus, June, 1971.

"Venereal disease. Communities strike back," by W. F. Schwartz. AM J NURS. 71:724, April, 1971.

"Venereal disease. TLC with the penicillin," by R. Mathews. AM J NURS. 71:720-723, April, 1971.

"The venereal disease dilemma: a case in question," by S. J. Bender. J SCH HEALTH. 41:105-107, February, 1971.

"Venereal disease: the enemy is us," by M. F. Doherty. NY STATE ED. 58:19-27, March, 1971.

"Venereal disease in women. I.," by C. S. Nicol. BR MED J. 2:328-329, May 8, 1971.

--II. by C. S. Nicol. BR MED J. 2:383-384, May 15, 1971.

"Venereal disease pandemic," by C. Roberts, et al. NY TIMES MAG. November 7, 1971, p. 62 plus.

"Venereal disease problem in Canada," by S. E. Acres, et al. CAN NURSE. 67:24-27, July, 1971.

"Venereal disease rampant." JAMA. 218:731, November 1, 1971.

"Venereal disease research; slow progress." CHEM & ENG N. 49:46-48 plus, June 21, 1971.

VENEREAL DISEASE

"Venereal diseases." BORD MED. 4:479-480, February, 1971.

"Venereal diseases." LANCET. 1:691-692, April 3, 1971.

"Venereal diseases at present," by W. Burckhardt. PRAXIS. 60:408-411, March 30, 1971.

"Venereal diseases in Lagos," by T. Daramola, et al. ISR J MED SCI. 7:288-294, February, 1971.

"Venereal diseases--new problems for the physician and the community," by A. J. Dalzell-Ward. DISEASE-A-MONTH. January, 1971, p. 1-45.

"Venereal infection." MIDWIFE HEALTH VISIT. 7:173, May, 1971.

"The X in sex." NURS TIMES. 67:380-381, April 1, 1971.

VULVITIS
"Salivary vulvitis," by B. A. Davis. OBSTET GYNECOL. 37:238-240, February, 1971.

YAWS
"Neuro-ophthalmological study of late yaws. I. An introduction to yaws," by J. L. Smith. BR J VENER DIS. 47:223-225, August, 1971.

--II. The Caracas project," by J. L. Smith, et al. BR J VENER DIS. 47:226-251, August, 1971.

"Osseous yaws and goundou," by L. Cornet, et al. J CHIR. 102:101-104, July-August, 1971.

"Test patterns of yaws antibodies in New Zealand," by A. Fischman, et al. BR J VENER DIS. 47:91-94, April, 1971.

YAWS

"Yaws," by I. Kantor, et al. ARCH DERMATOL. 103:546-547, May, 1971.

"Yaws, Mycoplasma pneumoniae and cold agglutinins in New Guineans," by P. B. Booth. MED J AUST. 1:715, March 27, 1971.

"Yaws, Mycoplasma pneumoniae and cold agglutinins in New Guineans," by J. Kariks. MED J AUST. 1:85-87, January 9, 1971.

YOUTH

"Cutaneous and venereal diseases seen at a drug-oriented youth clinic," by R. N. Richards. ARCH DERMATOL. 104:438-440, October, 1971.

"Juvenile progressive paralysis," by V. Satkova, et al. CESK PEDIATR. 26:500-501, October, 1971.

"Psycho-social aspects of venereal diseases in teen-agers," by I. Datt. INDIAN J DERMATOL. 16:27-35, January, 1971.

"Venereal disease in teen-agers," by H. M. Wallace. CLIN OBSTET GYNECOL. 14:432-441, June, 1971.

"Venereal diseases. A study of the attitudes toward and knowledge of them among young people," by J. Wallin. LAKARTIDNINGEN. 68:199-205, January, 1971.

AUTHOR INDEX

Abate, L., 20
Acosta, A. A., 37
Acres, S. E., 75
Adams, E. W., 10
Adkinson, N. F. Jr., 56
Akovbian, A. A., 61
Alarcon, C. J., 65
Allyn, G., 4
al-Salihi, F. L., 45
Alteras, I., 50
Amblard, P., 16, 17
Amman, R., 4
Amstey, M. S., 40
Anderson, J. R., 12
Andreoli, C., 14
Arap, S., 14
Arizaga Cruz, J. M., 36
Armand, P., 64
Arya, O. P., 55

Bafverstedt, B., 18
Baker, A. L., 39
Barnes, W. G., 56
Barr, J., 29, 57
Barton, F. W., 74
Bartunek, J., 17, 68
Bashmakova, M. A., 55
Bazanov, V. A., 16
Becerra-Garcia, A., 10
Beck, K. J., 15

Becker, H., 41
Belli, L., 58
Belonogova, N. A., 3
Bender, S. J., 1, 75
Benell, F. B., 47
Berger, U., 19
Berlin, S. I., 45
Bernfeld, W. K., 30, 33
Bharier, M. A., 12, 23, 33
Bhorade, M. S., 44
Bianchi, F., 70
Biehler, H., 64
Biemans, R., 58
Bienias, L., 20, 36, 58
Bierre, T. H., 74
Bilik, V. G., 42
Blanzaco, A., 72
Blaurock, G., 50
Boldt, I., 40
Bol'shakova, E. N., 22
Boneff, A. N., 52
Booth, P. B., 77
Bowszyc, J., 9, 55
Braff, E. H., 51
Bratkowa, A., 61
Bratus', N. V., 54
Braun, P., 9
Bredland, R., 17
Breen, R. M., 50
Brn, W. J., 74
Bro-Jorgensen, A., 29, 46

187

190

Potapnev, F. V., 6, 37
Prokop, A., 31
Pulchartova, E., 19
Pullen, H., 5

Quaife, R. A., 26
Quie, P. G., 4

Racouchot, J. E., 18
Racz, I., 58
Rambeck, W., 62
Randazzo, S. D., 55
Raszeja-Kotelba, B., 34
Ratnatunga, C. S., 25
Ravich, A., 76
Rawls, W. E., 28
Renoux, M., 49
Resl, V., Jr., 49
Reznichek, R. C., 31
Reznikova, L. S., 19
Reyn, A., 43
Richards, R. N., 18
Reising, G., 42
Rieth, H., 26
Riggs, M., 75
Ritzerfeld, W., 35
Rivoire, J., 5
Roberts, C., 75
Roberts, F. L., 68
Rodin, IuA., 25
Rodin, P., 67
Rodriguez, H. A., 38
Rodrigues, V., 72
Roitburd, M. F., 71
Rosebury, T., 1, 55
Rosener, F., 58
Rotmistrov, M. M., 6
Rouques, L., 17
Rowe, R. E., 56

Rozina, L. A., 50
Rubin, D., 74
Rubinchik, M. A., 13
Rudaev, V. A., 17
Rudolph, A. H., 53
Russo, E., 55
Ruszczak, Z., 50
Ruszel, K. B., 11
Rytel, M. W., 67

Sagdeeva, L. G., 46
Sanders, R., 30
Sartoris, S., 26
Satkova, V., 38
Sawazaki, C., 12
Scanlon, J. W., 20
Schachter, J., 15
Schenone, H., 35
Schmidt, H., 13
Schmor, J., 62
Schoch, E. P., Jr., 67
Schofield, C. B., 8, 29, 30
Schonebeck, J., 77
Schroeter, A. L., 8, 66
Schuppli, R., 66
Schwartz, W. F., 74
Schwarz, H., 4
Searle-Jordan, V. T., 59
Sefer, M., 52
Sehgal, V. N., 61
Seiga, K., 41
Selwyn, S., 9
Semenov, S. F., 7
Shannon, J. L., 67
Shapiro, L. H., 46
Sherlock, S., 39
Shetsiruli, L. T., 3
Shkliar, I. I., 68
Shore, W. B., 45
Silverman, M., 47

191

Vasil'ev, T. V., 12, 39, 70
Vejjajiva, S., 50
Verso, M. L., 66
Vesely, K., 60
Vidal, J., 65
Vincinti, N. H., 11
Vlasis, G., 68
Voisin, C., 26
Vojta, M., 76
Volter, D., 69
Vorobeichik, S. M., 51

Walker, A. N., 53
Walker, M., 31
Wallace, H. M., 75
Wallace, V. H., 51
Wallin, J., 76
Ward, M. E., 6, 50
Warrell, D. A., 49
Waugh, M. A., 7, 71
Weitgasser, H., 70
Wende, R. D., 73
Werko, L., 10

Werner, H. P., 37
West, B. S., 8
Westphal, A., 7
Westrom, L., 21
Wierer, A., 11
Wigfield, A. S., 73
Wilcox, R. R., 17, 69
Wilkinson, A. E., 34, 55
Wilkinson, R. H., 16
Williams, D. I., 72
Willman, K., 54
Wisniewski, H., 11
Wolin, L. H., 46
Wols-Van der Wielen, 57
Woodcock, K. R., 53
Worwag, Z., 36, 45
Wright, D. J., 63
Wright, J. M., 59

Yogeswari, L., 48
Yoshida, F., 41

Zablotniak, R., 60
Zavell, P. M., 48